A Doctor's Guide to Men's Private Parts

JAMES H. GILBAUGH, JR., M.D.

CROWN PUBLISHERS, INC.

NEW YORK

This book contains guidelines and instructions to be used
within the context of a personal health care program. The
instructions in this book are not intended as a substitute for
professional medical advice.

Published by Crown Publishers, Inc., 225 Park Avenue South,
New York, New York 10003.

CROWN is a trademark of Crown Publishers, Inc.

Manufactured in the United States of America

Library of Congress Cataloging-in-Publication Data

Gilbaugh, James H., Jr., M.D.
A doctor's guide to men's private parts.
Includes index.
1. Andrology—Popular works.   2. Generative organs,
Male.   I. Title.
RC881.G54   1988   612'.61   88-16226
ISBN 0-517-57138-2

10   9   8   7   6   5   4   3   2   1

First Edition

*This book is dedicated to
my wife, Marilyn, and to my family,
as well as to my teachers and patients*

CONTENTS

A Doctor's

Guide to

Men's

Private

Parts

INTRODUCTION

The same questions asked over and over by my patients led me to search for a book to help satisfy their curiosity. I found nothing in print that filled the bill, and this led to the creation of this book. It describes the private parts of a male's body and how those parts function. It details how they work separately and together, how they can go haywire, and whether they can be repaired or replaced. And to make the book accessible, I wrote it in basic, everyday, real-people language.

You have been urinating since birth and thinking nothing of it; it comes naturally. As you mature, you don't have to know anything about sex to experience it, for it too is one of nature's urges.

For most men, the dual yet separate function of the penis is performed for years without problems. But the aging process begins at birth, and as we grow older, parts weaken and malfunction: an erection fades or it doesn't happen at all; urine flow is restricted or blocked; blood appears in the semen or urine. Obviously, something is wrong when any of these things happen. The body has accumulated a bit of mileage. It's then that it is reassuring to have an idea about what may be happening and what you can do about it.

The drawing on page 2 identifies and locates the male private parts and accessories both inside and outside his body. The penis and the testicles are familiar, but the third organ, the prostate gland, is less so. All operate automatically when the brain sends down its signal. This efficient system ordinarily works well for years, but as men age the prostate gland may become enlarged, the

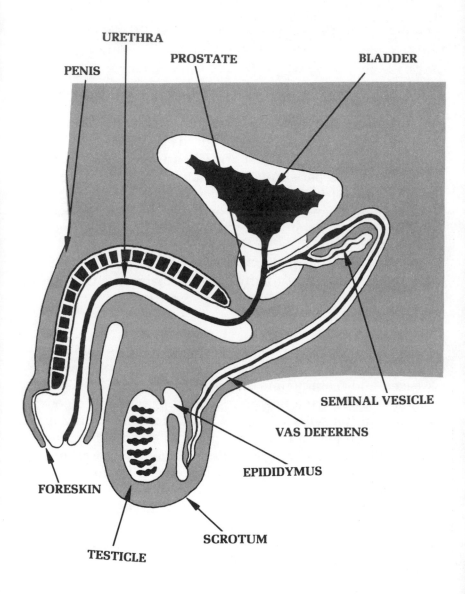

URETHRA

PROSTATE

BLADDER

PENIS

SEMINAL VESICLE

VAS DEFERENS

EPIDIDYMUS

FORESKIN

SCROTUM

TESTICLE

penis may fail to become erect, and the testicles may develop any number of problems.

Fortunately, most malfunctions can be repaired. Prostate obstruction can be relieved, artificial erections can be created, and most testicle problems can be treated. More in-depth discussions follow in the subsequent chapters.

In summary, this book describes for you the function of men's private parts and accessories. You will be able to recognize and anticipate potential problems and know when to seek appropriate repairs. In addition, trouble spots will be identified and solutions will be presented.

Chapter 10 presents the results of a lifestyle survey reporting the sexual expectations and experiences of a group of men, aged thirty-five to fifty years. Men, you should try the quizzes on pages 103 and 107 and compare results with the men I surveyed. Ladies, if you are interested in learning how men operate, you may be surprised when you read the results and comparisons.

The pages ahead are packed with clear, useful information. Men and women alike are invited to read on and make those private parts become familiar parts.

TROUBLE
SHOOTING

1

Problem 1: My penis isn't big enough.
   Answer: No man thinks his penis is big enough.
   Penis size has nothing to do with climax or
   orgasm. (See Chapter 3.)

Problem 2: It takes me longer to achieve an erection
   than when I was younger.
   Answer: Possibly. The firmest erections are reached
   during adolescence, the years of spontaneous erections. As a man ages beyond his
   thirties or forties, direct stimulation of the
   penis may be required to achieve erection.
   (See Chapter 3.)

Problem 3: My erections are not as stiff as they were
   when I was younger.
   Answer: This is often true. Hormones and blood vessels operate differently after teen years have
   passed. A certain reduction in stiffness may
   be expected. (See Chapter 3.)

Problem 4: I can't get one erection after another, as I
   once could.
   Answer: The "refractory period," the time it takes to
   get another erection after ejaculation and
   orgasm, increases with age. It is very brief
   for a teenager, but can be twenty-four hours

JAMES H. GILBAUGH, JR., M.D.

in later years. This is normal. (See Chapter 2.)

Problem 5: I lose my erection during sex more frequently than before.

Answer: Again, this may be a result of the aging process at work. Lack of concentration, distracting noises, fear of interruption, and other environmental influences—including your partner—can affect performance. (See Chapter 5.)

Problem 6: My penis requires more stimulation to reach orgasm.

Answer: Through the aging process, again, all things slow down. This includes sensitivity, nerve conduction, and blood vessel activity. More stimulation is needed as a man ages. (See Chapter 3.)

Problem 7: I will become impotent if I have a prostate operation.

Answer: Not true. Most prostate operations should not interrupt a man's ability to have an erection and successful intercourse. (See Chapters 2 and 7.)

Problem 8: Prostate operations are painful.

Answer: Not true. Most men fear this operation because they think it is very painful, but it isn't. The operation is usually performed under a spinal anesthetic, which allows complete consciousness without pain. (See Chapter 7.)

Problem 9: Isolated periods of impotence indicate impending doom.

Answer: Not true. Isolated episodes of impotence can

happen during sexual encounters at any age and are not unusual. These blank periods usually are associated with stressful situations, initial sexual encounters, or alcohol or drug overuse. (See Chapter 5.)

Problem 10: I am "done" if I fail to reach orgasm.
Answer: Not so. As a man ages, it is not uncommon to fail to reach orgasm during sex. It is also easier to get another erection if there was no ejaculation with the last one. (See Chapter 2.)

Problem 11: I ejaculate a smaller amount of semen than I once did.
Answer: True. A decrease in volume of ejaculate during intercourse is normal as a man ages. Older men, in their seventies and eighties, may not ejaculate at all but still have orgasms. (See Chapter 2.)

Problem 12: Ejaculation is not effective unless it is powerful.
Answer: Not true. In a man's prime, ejaculate can spurt two feet, but the process loses vigor as age affects muscle functions and nerve and blood supplies. (See Chapter 2.)

Problem 13: I'm afraid that masturbation when I was younger, or even now, may affect my sexual functioning in the future.
Answer: Nonsense. Lack of education and feelings of guilt promote myths of this sort. They have no basis in scientific fact. (See Chapter 2.)

Problem 14: Alcohol decreases my sexual ability.
Answer: Maybe. Alcohol in small amounts can stimulate interest in sex, but in larger amounts it

is a depressant and can cause impotence. (See Chapter 5.)

Problem 15: **As I get older, my penis gets smaller.**
Answer: Untrue. As you get older, your stomach gets fatter, so proportionately your penis looks smaller. No kidding; it's an optical illusion. (See Chapter 3.)

Problem 16: **If I have serious heart trouble—a heart attack or open cardiac bypass surgery—my sex life will be over.**
Answer: Not so. It is not necessary to forgo sexual activity after a heart attack; most men can resume sex without any serious effects. (See Chapter 5.)

Problem 17: **Masturbation makes me feel guilty.**
Answer: Masturbation is an important part of a person's sexuality. Men and women—married and single, young and old—do it. (See Chapter 2.)

Problem 18: **Will smoking reduce my sexual ability?**
Answer: Yes. Nicotine can constrict small blood vessels and has a dampening effect on a man's erectile ability—both immediate and long-term. (See Chapter 5.)

Problem 19: **Recreational drugs get me in the mood for sex, but they are dangerous.**
Answer: Marijuana, cocaine, and amphetamines can increase sexual desire and lower inhibitions in the short run, but over time can cause impotence and other serious hazards to health. (See Chapter 5.)

Problem 20: I have arthritis. Will sex help?
Answer: It might. Many patients find relief for four to six hours after having an orgasm. (See Chapter 2.)

Problem 21: My ulcer medication makes me impotent.
Answer: This is a common complaint among patients being treated for ulcers with certain drugs that block male hormone production as a side effect. (See Chapter 5.)

Problem 22: Blood pressure pills make me impotent.
Answer: Possibly. Medicines used to treat high blood pressure limit pressure required for an erection, so difficulties may result. (See Chapter 5.)

Problem 23: Is a person who tests negative for AIDS a safe sex partner?
Answer: Absolutely not. A negative test for HIV antibody is no guarantee that an individual cannot transmit AIDS. There is a lag time of six months or longer after infection occurs before the blood test shows positive. "Safe-sex clubs" won't prevent AIDS. (See Chapter 8.)

Problem 24: Can antibiotics prevent sexually transmitted diseases, including AIDS?
Answer: No. Antibiotics *cannot* prevent the HIV infection that causes AIDS, although oral antibiotics can prevent some other sexual diseases. Different diseases require different medications. Since there is no possible way to predict or cover every eventuality, it's a bad idea to gobble up an assortment of pills before every sexual adventure. (See Chapter 8.)

Problem 25: A vasectomy will cause hardening of the arteries, heart disease, or other diseases.

Answer: Not true. A study by the National Institutes of Health of 10,000 sterilized men found no increased risk of developing any such disorders. (See Chapter 2.)

EJACULATION, CONDOMS, AND VASECTOMY

2

On reaching puberty, a boy soon discovers that he can get an erection and that, with a little stroking, his erection can produce ejaculate. It is commonly called a "hard-on" and the sticky fluid that spurts out is called "come" or "cum."

Masturbation is usually the earliest form of adolescent experimentation with the mysteries of sex. It also is probably the scariest, because of its affiliation with temptation and evil in a vacuum of ignorance. No, it won't make you crazy or affect your adult sex life. Masturbation is the shock absorber of puberty, easing the bumps of adolescent development.

A boy's penis will become erect while he's asleep during the night. This is a nocturnal erection, a normal, automatic function. Frequently this erection will produce a nocturnal emission, called a "wet dream." That's okay, too. The wet dream is a cushion of adolescence that relieves pressure in a male body that produces semen that has no place to go.

> Maria, a nurse on our hospital day shift, raised five boys through their teens. She talked to me once about different reactions to nocturnal emissions, from boy to boy and time to time. The condition of their sheets after a wet dream

was evidence her sons feared would be discovered. One even washed his own sheets before his mother got up in the morning, to try to keep the secret from her.

When Maria talked to me, I assured her that nocturnal emissions were healthy indications of manhood, and that she ought to reassure her sons. She said later that the revelation that "Mom knows all about it and it's okay" ended her sons' guilt.

Most males have erections regularly through the night. This occurs from infancy through old age, so long as a man has the capability of erection. A normal, healthy man will have five erections during a night's sleep, spaced an hour to an hour and a half apart and lasting twenty to thirty minutes each. Usually the only evidence of all this activity is the erection a man finds when he awakens in the morning and feels a need to urinate. His bladder erection, or "piss hard-on," is actually his last erectile achievement of the night.

For a man in doubt, a test of whether or not he can still get an erection is to learn what happens at night. A simple but effective method is to tape postage stamps around his limp penis and see in the morning if the stamps have been separated by an erection. A more elaborate "snap gauge" is available commercially, but stamps will do as well.

Scientists have identified two kinds of sleep: dreaming sleep and nondreaming sleep. These alternate during the night; most men experience both kinds. During dreaming sleep, eyes move rapidly and eyeballs seem almost to jump. This is called REM sleep (for "rapid eye movement"). Most erections occur during REM sleep.

Nocturnal erections at an earlier age are more prevalent and are of longer duration, but as years pass they become shorter and fewer in number.

The amount of fluid men ejaculate and the force of its thrust decrease with age. Eventually, ejaculate may barely reach beyond the penis. But there are aberrations. In some cases, ejaculate doesn't come until after intercourse is completed; in other cases, it doesn't come at all.

The volume of fluid in each ejaculation varies, from 1.5 to 5 cubic centimeters. The average is 3 cc, about a teaspoonful. With age, volume peters out and sometimes disappears. The ejaculate squirts out in several whitish jellylike clumps. Very rapidly the gel is liquefied by an enzyme to an opaque watery fluid. This liquid form aids the sperm on its trip to the female egg for fertilization.

One of nature's anomalies is the wide variation of ejaculate volume produced among animals. A bull elephant produces a prodigious amount, as might be expected. He's good for more than 300 cc (more than a cup). A stallion produces 70 cc. But a man's production is well below the average production of a dog, 20 cc.

Contrary to common belief, testicles are not the major source of ejaculate. Seminal vesicles, small pouches behind the bladder and the prostate, produce about 70 percent of ejaculate volume; about one-third is produced by the prostate. Less than 1 percent is produced by the testicles, which do produce all sperm.

Among other minor contributors are Cowper's glands, paired pea-size glands directly below the prostate, which drain into the urethral tube. These were first identified by William Cowper in 1698. After almost three centuries, medical science still does not fully understand their function. However, one fact is certain: they produce drops of seminal fluid that appears at the head of the penis during sexual arousal but before ejaculation. These secretions often contain live sperm, so they add risk to the plan of withdrawal before ejaculation to prevent pregnancy.

Sperm cells are produced by the millions, from 40 million to 200 million per cubic centimeter (120 million to 600 million cells in each ejaculation).

EJACULATORY CONTROL

Normal ejaculation occurs simultaneously with orgasm. There are three principal forms of abnormal ejaculation: premature, retarded, and retrograde.

Coming too soon may be the least troublesome of these aberrations, but it is the most frustrating. Consider the guy who made a visit to a prostitute and came in a basin while she was washing his penis. Premature ejaculation can cause more serious problems for a couple if the woman hasn't become aroused before her mate's fire is out. The remedy usually comes with practiced patience, assisted by counseling if the prematurity persists. Sex counselors Masters and Johnson have suggested a "squeeze" technique to remedy the problem. Their proposition is that momentary squeezing of the penis conditions a man's response and delays or postpones his ejaculation.

The opposite problem, retarded ejaculation, happens less often but it does happen, particularly among older men. Psychological problems may result, but a more apparent effect is that a couple simply gets tired from having to work longer and harder.

Retrograde ejaculation differs from the other forms because it has nothing to do with timing and its effect is permanent. It happens when the opening from the bladder does not close during erection and semen spurts backward into the bladder. "Wrong-way" semen later is passed with urination. A test to ascertain ejaculation is to sample urine for sperm count after ejaculation.

Retrograde ejaculation frequently follows a prostatectomy. It can also result from injuries to nerves following bowel, pelvic, or colon surgery. Retrograde ejaculation may also be caused by diabetes or nerve diseases. Backward ejaculation may be an early sign of diabetes. A man can still climax and feel the effects, but a woman can't be fertilized. However, certain medications can reverse the problem temporarily.

Victor, aged seventy, had been sexually active prior to his prostate operation. He came in for his six-week postoperative checkup with the news that he could get erections but couldn't ejaculate. Victor's only problem was that he hadn't read the instruction sheet he got when he was discharged from the hospital.

It explained that he could expect normal intercourse and normal orgasm, but no ejaculation. As a matter of fact, it was Victor's wife who discovered his retrograde ejaculation. Some couples prefer it that way because it isn't as messy.

INFERTILITY

Infertility, the inability to reproduce, is more common than generally believed. A couple may be considered infertile if no pregnancy occurs after a year or two of unprotected intercourse (without use of contraceptive methods). Infertility is a problem in 10 to 15 percent of marriages. The husband, if he proves to be the source of the problem, may find that he is "shooting blanks" for one of several possible reasons, among them an ineffective sperm count, a complete absence of live sperm, or retrograde ejaculation.

ARTIFICIAL INSEMINATION

For a select group of patients, artificial insemination may be the best way to induce pregnancy because sperm that bypass the vagina may have better success in swimming up the fallopian tube and impregnating the female egg.

Electrically stimulated ejaculation, a technique developed for use on animals, is now being applied successfully to humans. A probe in the rectum can stimulate ejaculation, even in cases of spinal cord injuries where normal ejaculation would be impossible.

PAIN RELIEVER?

Some patients report that their arthritic pain is relieved for one to six hours after an orgasm. This may be because hormone releases cause something like "runner's high," or it may be that orgasm blocks pain receptors in the brain with a cortisone-like substance.

ABSTINENCE

Long-term abstinence or non-use of erections can create anxiety, but normal physical functioning should return to the male if all systems—vascular, neurovascular, and hormonal—are intact. However, postmenopausal women who have not had intercourse for an extended time are likely to have been affected by vaginal atrophy and constriction. Various treatments are available, but the most effective is a cooperative and patient partner.

CONDOMS

More than $200 million worth of condoms are sold in the United States each year, perhaps one-third of them to women. Their current popularity results from their proven efficiency in preventing transmission of sexually transmitted diseases.

The alarming epidemic of AIDS (acquired immunodeficiency syndrome) has stimulated interest in condoms because they offer almost assured protection from the human immunodeficiency virus (HIV), which causes AIDS. This virus is carried by body fluids (blood, semen, vaginal secretions) that leave one partner and enter vulnerable openings (vagina, anus, urethra) of the other. Condoms act as a barrier to transmission of body fluids.

The AIDS-induced revival of condoms, which had fallen from favor with the development of birth control pills, in effect has given condoms a second purpose. Condom packages once had a label that read, "Sold for the Prevention of Disease Only," but they were bought—in drugstores, barbershops, and men's-room vending machines—by men who wanted sex but not pregnant girlfriends. In those days they were call "rubbers." Now once again they are bought and sold as condoms for disease protection.

Used properly and consistently, condoms are 90 percent effective in preventing both pregnancy and sexually transmitted diseases.

A condom is a latex rubber sheath that rolls tightly over an erect penis. Also called a "prophylactic" or "skin," it is a modern version of a lambskin cecum (pouch) believed by many to have been invented in England in the eighteenth century by a Dr. Condom, although such a person may not have existed.

Some condoms still are made from membranes of animal intestines. They are especially comfortable, but their natural pores are not assured safe protection against virus penetration. Other condom materials have been introduced, but most have been manufactured from latex rubber since that process was introduced in the 1930s.

More than one hundred brands of condoms are made and sold in the United States. Most are seven or eight inches long and are rolled and packaged individually in plastic or foil. There are two principal design differences: some have reservoir ends to hold ejaculate and some do not; some are packaged in lubricant and some are not.

Condoms are also sold in assorted colors. They are available with "French tickler" and other end shapes, and with plain or ribbed sides, supposedly to increase sensitivity. Now condoms may be purchased with an adhesive ring that fits around the base of the penis to prevent the condom from slipping off if the erection subsides.

Condoms manufactured in the United States must meet federal specifications for material and labeling. The shelf life of a condom is two years; an expiration date should be stamped on the package.

VASECTOMY

Medical science has developed two more emission-control techniques, vasectomy and the sperm bank deposit.

Vasectomy is a simple, safe, and effective birth-control method that blocks the flow of sperm into the seminal fluid by surgically cutting the tube, or vas deferens, in the scrotum.

The operation most often is conducted in a doctor's office, requires only a local anesthetic, and can be completed in fifteen or twenty minutes. Pain usually is minimal and discomfort disappears after a day or two.

The operation is completely effective in almost all cases, but some time is required to clear sperm that had entered the body's distribution system before the operation. For this reason, the patient must return for sperm counts until an examination of semen, obtained by masturbation, shows that the sperm count is zero. Usually a

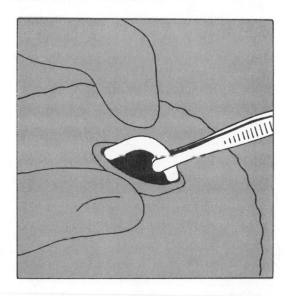

Vas deferens is identified through scrotal incision.

Both ends of the vas deferens are tied; at the option of the physician, the segment may or may not be removed.

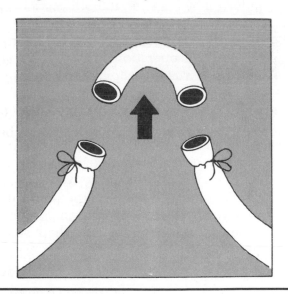

JAMES H. GILBAUGH, JR., M.D.

first check is made one month after the operation and another is made in two months.

Vasectomies are now performed on more than half a million men in the United States every year. It is safer than the more complicated tubal ligation, the comparable operation on a female.

After vasectomy, your manliness will not be affected. There is no effect on the male hormone produced by the testes. Your sexual functioning will not be altered. Your ability to have an erection and orgasm will not be changed, and the amount of semen ejaculated will not be noticeably decreased. Some patients say their sexual functioning is improved after vasectomy because the fear of unwanted pregnancy is relieved.

Before a vasectomy is performed, however, it is critical that the patient determine that he wishes to father no more children. The operation is intended to be irreversible. The patient should consider the possibilities of divorce and remarriage, however improbable they might seem to be. The operation must be authorized by the patient and endorsed by his wife, in both cases by written statements.

Recently, reversals of vasectomy have been performed with some success. An operation to rejoin the vas deferens tubes, called a *vasovasostomy*, has attracted the interest of men who have changed their minds. This operation is more complex and more expensive than the original vasectomy, and results are mixed. A high percentage of men who have had the operation have delivered sperm, but the pregnancy rate is about 50 percent, depending in part on the fertility of the woman.

Another way to preempt the permanency of a vasectomy is to store sperm before the operation. Frozen sperm banks are becoming more popular, but their success in inducing pregnancy remains to be seen.

Infertility

Fertility problems in men are related to the production, quality, and movement of male sperm. If infertility threatens to become a problem, there are hazards to avoid or factors to consider:

- **Coffee** *Medications with caffeine and coffee appear to make sperm sluggish and slow.*

- **Alcohol** *Too much alcohol lowers production of testosterone, a critical male sex hormone.*

- **Smoking** *Tobacco smoke lowers sperm count and slows sperm motility.*

- **Drugs** *"Recreational drugs," including marijuana, may decrease testosterone levels.*

- **Jeans** *Tight jeans or shorts can overheat sperm-producing cells in testicles, lowering sperm count.*

- **Hot tubs** *Frequent tub use also can lower sperm count by overheating sperm-producing cells.*

- **Age** *Sperm production drops sharply after thirty but can persist at lower levels into the nineties.*

- **Cimetidine** *This drug, prescribed for treatment of ulcers, also decreases testosterone level.*

- **Diethylstilbestrol** *This drug, used thirty to forty years ago to prevent miscarriages, was later found to cause fertility problems among men born to mothers using it.*

- **Vaginal douches** *Douches, sprays, and lubricants can immobilize sperm if certain chemicals are present.*

- **Infection** *All sexually transmitted diseases can affect fertility adversely.*

- **Diabetes** *Nerve and vascular damage created by diabetes can cause retrograde ejaculation so that sperm is not delivered.*

Tips on Condom Use

1. Don't use an old condom. Condoms have a safe shelf life of two years; they should have an expiration date stamped on the package. Don't stretch your luck.

2. Condoms are highly effective in blocking sexually transmitted diseases, but they are not foolproof. Remember, an uncovered herpes sore can bypass a condom.

3. Proper and consistent use of condoms is 90 percent effective in preventing pregnancy.

4. Proper and consistent use of condoms is required for prevention of sexually transmitted diseases.

5. To use a condom effectively:
   a. Place the correct side of the condom against the head of the penis. You'll know it's the wrong side if it won't unroll.
   b. Unroll the condom over an *erect* penis from head to base; allow a one-half-inch space at the front if there is no reservoir.
   c. Use the condom prior to foreplay, before the penis touches the vagina, mouth, or rectum.
   d. After ejaculation, remove the condom before the erection wilts; avoid spilling contents.

6. Use only a water-base lubricant (such as K-Y Jelly) with a condom; a petroleum base (such as Vaseline) may damage sensitive latex material.

7. Never use a condom more than once.

8. Keep condoms cool; do not store them in a wallet or glove compartment.

9. Don't be bashful about buying condoms.

10. Don't fill them with water and drop them from hotel room windows.

How to Use a Condom

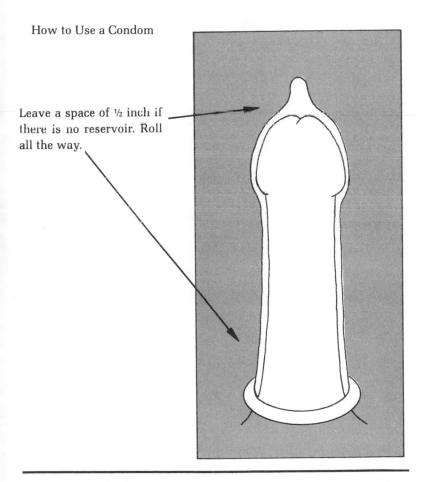

Leave a space of ½ inch if there is no reservoir. Roll all the way.

T H E
P E N I S

3

The penis is a complex organ. Blood pumped from all over the body contributes to an erection, or hard-on, in three steps: nerve stimuli causes the wall muscles of tiny penile blood vessels to relax and to accommodate a greater blood volume in the organ; blood under pressure fills the penis until it is stiff and erect; once filled, the penis traps the blood inside to maintain the erection. Blood volume is six to eight times the normal flow to the penis. Any malfunction of the nerves or blood vessels serving the penis can cause an erectile problem.

Three tubes that run the length of the penis engorge with blood to give erectness and stiffness. Two of them, spongy tubes called *corpora cavernosa*, absorb most of the blood. Some goes to a third tube, the *corpus spongiosum*, the covering of the urethra. (The urethra is the tube that runs through the penis and carries semen and urine.)

The product of this process, the size of an erection, is the most frequently expressed concern of men. Most wish they were bigger. Male erections generally range from four and a half inches to eight inches, but most are six inches. Minor bends in the penis are not uncommon and do not interfere with function. They are technically called *chordee*. Surgery may be necessary to correct severe chordee.

Some helpful statistics were provided by an enterpris-

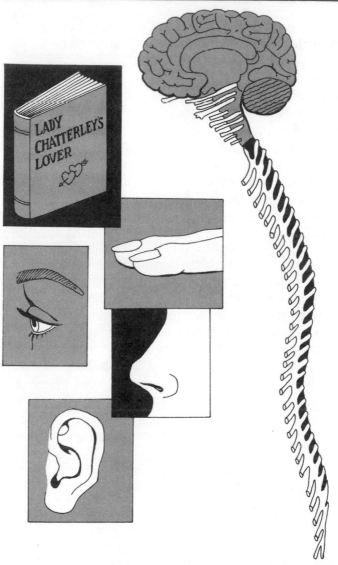

The making of an erection—The brain is probably the largest sex organ in man. Many elements, including psyche, touch, sight, smell, and hearing, are important for initiating and maintaining an erection. Some think that smell is the most important, but this is debatable.

ing lady who worked in a massage parlor. She put the tape to the erections of 1,681 of her customers, presumably as part of her warm-up routine, and published her findings in *Playboy*. Her research indicated that 97 percent of the men she measured achieved the average six inches; only seven of the 1,681 came up to eight inches.

A fact that men are reluctant to accept is that penis size is not proportionate to sexual satisfaction for either male or female. Nature placed the sensual nerve endings that facilitate orgasm at the most practical place possible, up front: on a man they are at the head of his penis (glans penis); on a woman they are at a protrusion above the opening of the vagina (clitoris). Stimulation, not depth of thrust, is all that is needed.

> *Alex, a fifty-four-year-old photographer, confided that all his life he had been bothered because his penis was too small. He said that even with a full erection he couldn't get a condom to stay on unless he first wrapped a tissue around his penis. I assured him that no matter what the size (agreeing silently that his penis was indeed small), it was big enough to have intercourse.*
>
> *Hundreds of times I've heard men complain about the sizes of their penises, but never because it was too big. This case shows that sometimes, regardless of what a doctor says, the patient might be right.*

CIRCUMCISION

Circumcision is surgical removal of the foreskin that covers the head of the penis. The operation is usually performed shortly after birth. The practice dates back to 4000 B.C. among tribal cultures in several parts of the world, and now is performed for religious or medical reasons.

In modern Western culture, its practice by members of the Judaic religion symbolizes Abraham's covenant with God: "Every male among you shall be circumcised. You shall be circumcised in the flesh of your foreskins, and it shall be a sign of the covenant between me and you." (Genesis 17:10–11)

In the United States, circumcision is a fairly routine procedure for nonreligious reasons. The custom is much less prevalent in Europe, although few operations are based on medical opinion. Medical opinion, in fact, is undecided about the use of circumcision for health reasons.

Debate on the relationship between circumcision and cancer is a pendulum of diverse opinions. Nevertheless, the fact remains that the great majority of penile cancer victims were not circumcised at birth. It seems reasonable to suggest circumcision as a precaution against such a devastating disease.

There is some agreement on medical issues concerning circumcision:

- There is no proof that circumcision protects against venereal disease.
- There is conflicting evidence regarding cancer of the cervix in sexual partners of uncircumcised men.
- Circumcision may prevent penile cancer. Proper retraction of foreskin with cleansing of the penis is also a means of prevention.
- In young boys, there is a significant increase in urinary-tract infections in those who are not circumcised.
- Meatitis (inflammation of the opening of the urethra) and meatal stenosis occur more frequently in circumcised boys.

■ Injuries from circumcision are rare but do occur and vary from minor to severe. Occasionally the penis will require an additional procedure to correct the injury.

The operation is a simple excision of the foreskin. Infection, should it occur, can easily be treated with an antibiotic ointment. Significant injury to the penis itself is rare.

PROBLEMS

Impotence The absence of erectile function is the most common and most disturbing sexual problem among men. For years the reasons for impotence were thought to be psychological—"it's all in the mind"—but the influence of physical factors is becoming more and more evident. Alcohol is one factor that can cause problems that go beyond one night's failure. Smoking is another. Diabetes can cause impotence, even at an early age, because the disease damages nerves and blood vessels. Because of its commonness and complexity, impotence is the subject of a separate section of this book. (See Chapter 5.)

Although impotence is the most pervasive problem that can arise, there are others as well. Here are some:

Penile injury The penis itself can be injured during intercourse, usually when it thrusts abruptly against the pubis or pubic bone. Swelling, bleeding, and sometimes deformity of the penis can result.

An erect, inflexible penis can be injured in sexual activity. The penile urethra also can be permanently damaged by plastic swizzle sticks, ballpoint pens, hatpins, or other objects stuck in it to stimulate sensation.

A college student literally "broke it off" in his girlfriend when she was straddling him during vigorous intercourse. As he thrust deeply into her, she suddenly fell backward, bending his erect penis inside her. Both heard a pop. The suspensory ligament of the penis was broken, causing internal bleeding. This fellow didn't go to a hospital for two days, too late for effective surgical repair. As a consequence, his penis was permanently deformed and from then on he was unable to achieve normal erections. Penile injury should be treated by a doctor immediately.

Peyronie's disease This is sometimes described as "bent spike" because the erect penis actually bends in the middle, or anywhere along the shaft, and angles upward, downward, or to one side. The effect is caused by a small lump of plaque, which feels like gristle, at the point of the bend. Peyronie's disease most often occurs in the fourth or fifth decade of life, although it has developed in teenagers and in men over eighty.

A carpenter, aged fifty-five, came in with a fear of cancer. He had a lump near the top of his penis, and for the past three months his erections bent at that point and were painful. The erections were no longer full, but looked like an hourglass, as though blood was not getting through. When this man tried intercourse, his penis bent back on itself.

I prescribed vitamin E, but perhaps helped most by reassuring him that the condition was not cancer and that it disappears or softens in one-third of patients without treatment. In three months his pain was gone and he could have intercourse—but carefully, because his shaft was still bent slightly.

Although Peyronie's disease is a relatively common problem from teen years on, its cause remains unknown. No effective remedy is known, but vitamin E seems to help. Patients also can be relieved of anxiety with assurance that the growth is not cancerous. Surgical removal has been attempted, but the most effective surgery is implantation of a penile prosthesis in severe cases.

Balanitis This is an inflammation of the foreskin and underlying tissues at the head of the penis, where, in uncircumcised men, a natural secretion can collect. The condition can be caused by friction from damp clothing, chemicals in clothing fabrics, or a reaction to various contraceptives. Some men are allergic to vaginal jellies and creams or to lubricants in condoms. The effect is a reddening and irritation of the penis. The easiest solution in these cases is to change jellies or condoms.

A teacher, aged thirty-eight, complained of recurring inflammation on the head of his penis, and of tight foreskin, which he had treated in the past with salves. His problem was resolved by a circumcision, performed on an outpatient basis with local anesthetic.

This was a case where circumcision for hygienic purposes was appropriate. Recurrent problems with infection, such as with this patient, who was a diabetic, require surgery.

Phimosis This condition makes it difficult to retract a tightened foreskin off the penile head. The hood won't go up. Phimosis is caused by chronic infection, but may be congenital. Circumcision may be necessary for cure.

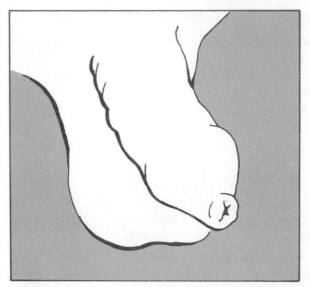

Phimosis

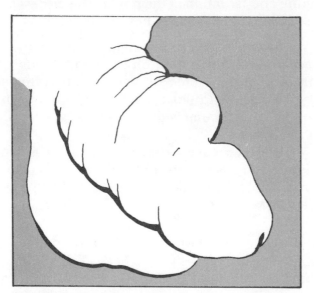

Paraphimosis with edema

*Sam, aged sixty-seven, a lawyer, hadn't seen
the head of his penis for years. When he came
into the examining room, the penis was foul-
smelling and inflamed. I could not pull the
foreskin back to examine the head. Circumcision was necessary to relieve the conditions,
and in that process I found a cancer, confirmed
by biopsy.*

Paraphimosis This condition, caused by infection or
trauma, prevents a tightened foreskin from going back
over the head of the penis. It is stuck behind the head; the
hood won't go down. Tightened like a constricting ring
around the penis, it produces swelling, which then produces more swelling.

*Paul, a thirty-eight-year-old realtor, appeared
in my office with a gigantic, swollen penis. The
foreskin had gotten stuck behind the head of the
penis during what Paul claimed was a midafter-
noon business meeting in a local motel.*

*His penis had swollen to three or four times
its normal size while he was "doing business";
it looked like a glazed doughnut. I relieved the
pressure by lubricating the head of the penis
and pushing it back through the ring, something like slipping a tight ring off a finger. Later
I made permanent cure possible with a circumcision.*

Urethral stricture This condition is a narrowing of the
urethral tube in one or several places, which restricts
urine flow. In concept, it is similar to a long tunnel with
what appears to be a very constricted opening at the far
end. A urethral stricture usually is caused by infection or
trauma, but sometimes it is congenital in origin. Its signs

are a slow, weak urine flow and, sometimes, weakened expulsion of seminal fluid or urethral discharge.

Urethral strictures may be single or multiple and may appear in various places within the urethra, from the tip of the penis to the area of the prostate. Treatment may be either dilating the tube or cutting it in the appropriate places with a special instrument.

Priapism This is a case of a persistent erection and might seem to be the ultimate among male fantasies. It isn't; in fact, it can cause permanent damage. Priapism produces an erection even in the absence of sexual stimulation, or it maintains an erection after intercourse, because engorged blood that created the erection cannot flow back by general circulation through the body. Its cause usually is a red blood cell disease or injury to the spinal cord. It should be treated immediately—which means a visit to a hospital emergency room or a doctor's office. If the condition can be corrected quickly by medication or irrigation of the penis, normal erectile functions probably will be regained. Otherwise, surgery may be necessary.

An erection that won't go away after ejaculation and intercourse is abnormal. Priapism also may follow injections to initiate erections. (See Chapter 5.) Immediate medical attention is essential, but even with immediate treatment, impotence may result.

Skin problems Like the owner of a new car who notices every nick and scratch, a man will examine his penis for minute aberrations. Blackheads—and whiteheads, too—commonly show on the underside of the penis, although they can form on any part of penile skin. These little devils are more of a nuisance than anything else. They are caused by plugged glands or ducts, and may be easily popped out, but they probably will reappear.

Rashes and moles likewise are common, and may cause

no problems. A doctor can tell whether skin problems are significant, such as symptoms of balanitis, or are harmless.

Drips after urination   There is an inescapable truth in the old verse that goes, "No matter how you jump and dance, the last few drops go in your pants." It's a circumstance called postmicturitional dribbling, and that's the way it is.

> Here's an experiment you can conduct yourself. After voiding, apply gentle upward pressure under the base of the penis. In most cases the pressure will release those last few drops.

Bites   Bites on the penis, whether from a playful sex partner or a dangerous insect, should receive prompt medical attention.

> A hunter at a deer camp in the hills was bitten on the penis while using an outhouse. At first the bite felt like a pinprick, but within hours the bite area became stiff and intensely painful. Soon the hunter experienced chills, fever, sweating, nausea, and severe abdominal pain. Fortunately a doctor was in the camp, and treated the victim with antivenin for what he recognized as a black widow spider bite. The hunter recovered fully.

Of more than 30,000 species of spiders in the world, fifty are known to bite humans. Two that are deadly are named by their colors, black widow and brown recluse. Unfortunately, both frequent residential and recreational areas. The black widow, an aggressive spider that will attack on slight provocation, spins its web in darkened places—including outhouses.

Penile trauma Because the penis is flexible and is in a reasonably protected location, serious injuries are unusual. But they do occur. Injury can be caused by such obvious sources as missiles, bullets, knives, blunt instruments, and burns, and such unconventional sources as a chain saw or the power takeoff on a hay machine.

> On a recent trip to Bangkok, I learned of a unique case of penile injury and repair. A soldier's ex-wife had severed his penis, and surgeons replaced it with a penis that was removed from a transsexual during a sex-change operation. The replacement penis grew into its new place nicely. It also greatly improved its new owner's outlook on his future. As far as I know, the operation was the first penile transplant in the world.

Foreign bodies Young men, especially preteen boys, experiment with their erections and consequently appear in emergency rooms with a bewildering array of objects stuck inside. I have removed pencils, pens, ladies' hatpins, and straight pins from inside young penises.

It is not unusual for a man or boy to catch his penis in his pants zipper, causing injury to the skin. I also have repaired skin damage caused by applying the business end of a vacuum cleaner tube to an erection, presumably to assist masturbation.

> A fifteen-year-old boy inserted a pencil up his urethra while masturbating, and the next thing he knew the pencil was gone. An X ray found the pencil in the bladder. I removed it through the normal channel—the way it went in.

In addition to insertion of foreign objects, penile injuries also are caused by experimentation from without.

Emergency-room physicians occasionally must remove rings that were rolled onto a penis in its relaxed state and then stuck tight after erection because blood could not escape. Among the bizarre objects I have seen hanging from a penis is a monkey wrench; the patient's penis was trapped through the hole in the handle.

T H E
T E S T I C L E S

4

esticles are an obvious and sensitive part of a man's sex system. Although they are conspicuous, at least in the locker room, they are usually not a cause for self-consciousness, as penis size may be. Even a casual look reveals that one testicle hangs lower than the other. Nobody knows why, but the difference is perfectly normal. Neither is there reason for concern because one testicle is slightly larger or smaller than the other.

Some men are concerned, however, about whether their underwear might affect their fertility. There is some validity in this. Snug shorts, in addition to creating uncomfortable entanglements once in a while, draw the testicles closer to the body, raising internal testicle temperature slightly. This change can reduce sperm count and, in some men, reduce fertility.

The testicles are a source of sperm—the source of life itself—and of a male hormone, testosterone, which creates such masculine effects as facial hair and deep voices. Testicles are literally the "balls" associated with masculinity.

Early one Saturday morning, I received a phone call from my longtime friend Tom. In a distinctly frightened voice, he said he had three

> balls. I told him that that was impossible. To calm his worry, we met at my office for an examination. He had a spermatocele, a benign growth. It was located alongside his normal testicle, and I had to admit that it did look like a "third ball." These growths are usually noted on self-examination and are benign. They only need to be observed periodically or if they become painful or enlarge rapidly. They can be surgically removed if they become bothersome.
>
> I told my friend Tom that the growth wouldn't go away by itself, but that it was nothing to worry about and there was no need to operate. It's still there, a year later. I told Tom we might pick up some change at a bar, betting we had five balls between us, but he failed to enjoy my humor.

Each testicle is about two inches long and a bit more than an inch wide. As mentioned earlier, it is possible that one might be bigger or smaller than the other, but size does not affect function. Each has two types of cells where elements essential to sexual functioning are manufactured. One type manufactures sperm, the male seed; the other creates testosterone, a hormone.

A sperm cell transfers genetic characteristics through chromosomes. It swims through the reproductive channels of the male and later the female by swishing its tail back and forth. The testicles produce sperm in astronomical numbers, literally billions every year, although only one single sperm is needed for reproduction.

Men produce sperm continually from puberty throughout life, unlike women, who cease ovulation (the release of eggs) after menopause. If sperm aren't released through ejaculation, they die in the productive chain, but they are continually replaced.

After being produced in *seminiferous tubes* in the testicle, sperm cells move slowly through the *epididymis*, a microscopic network of coils behind the testicle. The trip takes about ninety days, the length of the sperm maturation process. Having matured, sperm cells swim through another tube, the *vas deferens*, pairs of which run from the testicle along and behind the bladder. These join at the *seminal vesicles*, pairs of glands that produce seminal fluid, and from the prostate are ejaculated, with semen, through the urethral tube in the penis.

It is possible to analyze semen to determine the presence and potency of sperm. This is a fertility test usually requested after a couple has been unable to achieve pregnancy after a year or so. Computer evaluation of a laboratory sample of semen can determine quantitatively the volume, density, and motility of sperm, all factors in fertility. Two or three analyses over six to eight weeks usually are necessary to determine a correct pattern.

Testosterone hormones produced by another type of cell in the testicle, called *Leydig's cells*, immediately enter the bloodstream for distribution throughout the body to serve their intended purposes. Testosterone is essential for sperm production and influences sexual aggression, sexual attraction, ability to obtain an erection, and potency. But unlike sperm, production of testosterone diminishes with age after peaking in the late teens.

It is estimated that more than 200 hormones are produced in the human body. Of all these, testosterone is known as the "male hormone" because of its exclusively male functions; estrogen is a comparable "female hormone" because its function is to maintain the condition of the vagina, including vaginal lubrication. Actually, both of these hormones are produced by both sexes, although in appropriately proportionate quantities.

A man can live quite nicely with just one testicle, whether the other was lost through an accident or an operation or was absent at birth, as sometimes happens. With one testicle, a man's sperm and hormone production can be normal and he need have no related concerns about performing sexually or fathering children.

A man's testicles have a cover, which is what shows outside. This is the *scrotum*, a sack with a compartment for each testicle; these compartments are separated by a *septum*, which acts as a "fire wall." The scrotum's most important function is protection of the testes and temperature control. Testicles are cooler than the rest of the body by one or two degrees, a temperature more favorable for the manufacture of sperm. The scrotum delicately controls temperature by muscles within its walls which raise the testicles when outside temperatures are cool (moving them closer to the body) and lowers them when outside temperature is warmer. The *spermatic cord*, to which each testicle is attached like a yo-yo, also has muscles which help in this movement. In combination, they're a built-in climate-control system.

Muscles of the scrotum wall also tighten at times of sexual arousal, perhaps as a protective device.

The up-front position of testicles makes self-examination simple, and periodic examination is a good habit to develop. The best time is while taking a warm shower or bath because the scrotum is relaxed at those times. Each testicle should feel like a hard-boiled egg with the shell removed. There should be no hard spots or lumps. Evidence of even painless lumps that feel hard should be reported to a physician immediately.

> *A graduate student had read about self-examination of testicles. He tried it and found a pea-sized bump on his right testicle. Two days later he was in my office. I saw right away that the growth was cancerous and removed it the next day. There were no signs that it had*

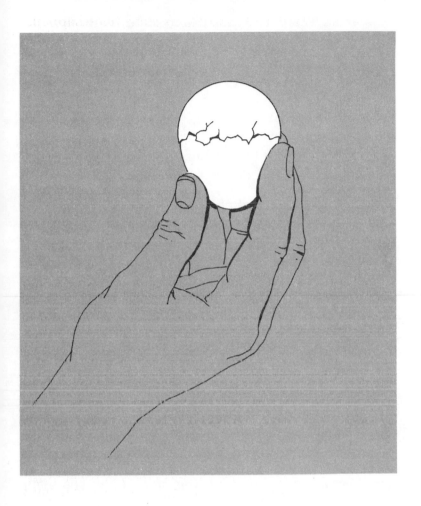

A normal testical should feel like a hard-boiled egg without the shell.

spread. This was a case where self-examination found a cancer early, so a cure was possible.

All the conditions below are abnormalities of the testicles and indicate a need to see a doctor.

Undescended testicles   Normally, testicles develop within the abdomen and descend just before birth or soon afterward. If one has descended improperly or incompletely, repair should be made by early childhood.

Twisted testicles   A testicle hangs from the spermatic cord like the clapper of a bell. Twisting and untwisting, or intermittent torsion on the cord, can occur during normal physical activity or even while sleeping. The condition most often occurs in young males, but not exclusively. Emergency surgery is recommended if the cord does not untwist.

Varicoceles   In this condition, veins in the spermatic cord enlarge and feel like a bag of worms. The condition is common in the mid-teens and usually is felt near the left testicle and cord. The bag of worms usually collapses when the patient is lying down. The feeling is uncomfortable, and the presence of varicoceles sometimes can cause a low sperm count.

Inguinal hernia   A rupture on the side of the spermatic cord in the groin causes a bulge that is most noticeable when a man has been standing quite a while. It may be painful and can strangulate bowels if trapped. The swelling usually goes down or disappears when the patient is lying down. A doctor should be consulted.

Appendix testis   This is a small growth attached to the testicle that can become inflamed or twisted, causing severe pain, tenderness, and swelling. Surgical removal is the usual cure.

Hydrocele   This is a collection of fluid surrounding the testicle, like a water balloon. The size varies with the volume of fluid. This condition can usually be diagnosed with a flashlight; it can be remedied by a simple surgical excision if it becomes bothersome.

Epididymitis   An inflammation of the epididymis caused by bacteria or virus. Swelling and pain often are accompanied by fever and chills. These are tender, hot balls.

Spermatocele   A cystic, grapelike mass containing enlarged sperm tubes near the epididymis causes concern because of its abnormal growth. It is not cancerous.

Orchitis   Inflammation of the testicles that produces painful swelling and usually is associated with mumps, and sometimes with epididymitis. Shrinkage of the testicles may occur after the disease clears.

Cancer   Most tumors of the testicle are cancerous, and most develop between the ages of fifteen and forty. It is a relatively rare cancer in other age groups. If the tumor is cancerous, the testicle is hard and may be swollen, but the lump or swelling usually is painless. The cancer may be very small. All these signs may be determined by self-examination. Any abnormality should be reported to a doctor immediately, because 90 percent of testicular cancers can be cured.

I M P O T E N C E

5

Impotence, the inability to achieve an erection and follow through with normal intercourse, occurs with surprising frequency as men age. An estimated ten million men in the United States are impotent.

There are degrees of impotence. Almost every man experiences temporary, or situational, impotence from an assortment of causes—too much to drink, mental preoccupation, lack of interest from his partner. This inhibition is easily explained and soon overcome. Lasting impotence is caused by more complex factors.

> *A forty-five-year-old fellow who successfully lured a lady to bed the night he met her was embarrassed because he couldn't get an erection no matter how hard both tried. He apologized, saying he guessed that he was over the hill. The attitude and condition improved substantially when he and his new friend got to know each other better and were more relaxed. This is an illustration of performance anxiety.*

Until very recently, impotence was blamed almost exclusively on psychological problems. Fifteen or twenty years ago, doctors thought mental concerns were responsible for 95 percent of impotence cases. The remaining 5 percent were attributed to evident physical causes such as obvious nerve damage.

Now doctors believe causes of impotence are almost equal between psychological and physical factors. The shift in emphasis is based on better diagnostic methods and on discoveries made possible by more sophisticated measurement of physical and chemical changes. In turn, these developments may be attributed to a new interest in scientific sex pioneered by Dr. Alfred Kinsey in the 1940s and 1950s. After Kinsey, researchers began looking where they had not looked before.

Both physical and psychological causes of impotence may be treated and, to a considerable extent, corrected, sometimes in dramatic fashion. Listed below are dominant physical and psychological causes, with some evidence of their effects.

PHYSICAL IMPOTENCE

Drugs

A fellow doctor found that he had become impotent and came to me for help. At the time he was treating himself for ulcers with the drug cimetidine. That was a clue; the drug is quite effective as a medication for ulcers, but it also may lower production of testosterone, a male hormone. His complaint of impotence was typical among users of that drug. I recommended a substitute medication, and the impotence problem disappeared.

Chemicals are the most common physical cause of impotence, and some provide surprises. Other medications with side effects related to impotence include high blood pressure pills (antihypertensives), which inhibit blood pressure for an erection; recreational drugs (marijuana, cocaine, amphetamines), which affect the central nervous system; antihistamines, such as cold pills; tranquilizers; weight-loss pills; diuretics; and sedatives.

Among the most frequent causes, alcohol abuse can have a more lasting impact than one night's disappointment; nicotine from cigarette smoking can cause impotence by constricting small blood vessels, limiting blood supply to the penis, as well as elsewhere throughout the body.

Abnormal Blood Pressure

A retired insurance executive, aged seventy, complained that his capacity to achieve an erection had been diminished after a coronary bypass operation and he could never get hard enough to penetrate. He said it was like trying to put an oyster in a parking meter. His problem was permanently decreased blood flow, and the best solution was implantation of a penile prosthesis—an artificial stiffener.

Because blood rushes into the penis to create an erection, obstruction of the blood vessels can result in impotence. High blood pressure, hardening of the arteries, Peyronie's disease, and diabetes are among diseases that can clog the fuel line. A new technique for measuring blood pressure in the penis also can confirm whether pressure there is abnormally low among some men who smoke.

Nerve Impulse Abnormalities

A forty-two-year-old man suffering from diabetes was also suffering from a sex problem too embarrassing, he thought, to take to a doctor in his own city. He had not had an erection for more than a year, but he could ejaculate while masturbating, often with his wife's participation.

He traveled 200 miles to consult me. The diabetes had speeded his aging process by affecting both his nerves and his blood vessels. We worked together to control his diabetes, but the cure was a penile prosthesis.

Nerves that control the penis are as essential to an erection as is blood. Diseases that can reduce or interrupt critical nerve impulses include strokes, spinal cord injuries, kidney disease, diabetes, and alcoholism. Nerve injuries from abdominal or pelvic surgery, or other causes, also inhibit nerve functions.

Hormonal Abnormalities

Richard, a fifty-nine-year-old impotent patient of mine was found to have a very low level of testosterone. He was suffering from a disease of the liver called hemochromatosis. The proper testosterone level was restored by injections. The patient eventually could get erections and claimed an increase in his sexual desire.

Impotence is rarely caused by an imbalance of hormones, but kidney and liver diseases, kidney dialysis, and alcoholism can adversely affect normal hormone balance.

PSYCHOLOGICAL IMPOTENCE

Depression

Nick, a security guard, had not wanted a divorce, but his wife left him for his best friend and took their four children with her. After she left, Nick's depression deepened and his potency failed altogether. He visited a psychiatrist regularly for a year, after which he felt more at ease psychologically but got no help in getting an erection.

Nick found a new girlfriend and dated her for a year that included a delightful trip to Hawaii. But she left him because he was incapable of getting an erection.

When he came to me, at age fifty, he had been divorced three years and no longer had a girlfriend. His routine included weekly visits to a massage parlor for fellatio, which brought him to ejaculation, but without erection. He was suffering from depression and performance anxiety.

However, he did awaken with a morning "piss hard-on," so I was able to convince him that his erection mechanism still worked.

Mental depression can tax a man's sex drive as well as his energy. Inability to achieve an erection leads to further depression and thus a vicious cycle.

Stress

A travel agent, aged forty-four, was typical of many patients. He was considering divorce, a possibility enthusiastically encouraged by a *girlfriend who listened eagerly to his talk about exotic trips together. The woman was much younger than the man, and he wished to impress her with his sexual performance. But he soon learned he wasn't the sexual sensation that he used to be.*

Actually, he wasn't capable of performing as he thought he used to. He forgot that the brain is a sex organ (the biggest of them all), and he was bombarding it with visions that were more than he could handle.

Problems with job, marriage, or money can easily become problems with sex. Inability to get an erection provokes stress, and a vicious cycle ensues.

Performance Anxiety

A fairly well-known lawyer could have intercourse with his alcoholic wife—but he didn't enjoy it. He preferred taking a girlfriend to his mountain cabin. However, the secluded location, the fireside, the music, and the wind in the trees unfortunately did him no good. He couldn't get an erection. He tried different women, same cabin with the romantic accessories, and still could have no erection.

He confided to me that he felt like somebody was trying to tell him something. I suggested he go to a marriage counselor, and the counselor did tell him something: "Go back to your wife." His wife, too, went to a counselor for alcoholism therapy. They're both back on a one-way street.

Jack, a twenty-eight-year-old bricklayer, could have normal intercourse except when he tried to put on a condom. Each time he tried to roll on a rubber, his erection faded. Obviously this was a psychological problem.

Persistent failure to achieve an erection, for whatever reason, can become self-perpetuating. Fear of failure is reinforced by failure.

Misinformation

A young man came in with a problem many men would like to have. He could make love to his girlfriend once a night easily, but he thought he should be able to do it three or four times. Was something wrong?

Well, there was something missing if this fellow wanted to be like the pro football player who bragged that he could make it with five women a day, except on game days. But for mere mortals, once a night consistently is average.

Misinformation about sex begins as soon as boys are old enough to discover there are differences between boys and girls. It takes adult forms, too, in myths about how a "real man" should perform, how a woman should react, how hope is lost with old age. Most men aren't as "real" as they'd like to believe they are, and, like cars, they peter out as age progresses.

There is a more serious side to misinformation. Statistics show that men who have had coronary bypass surgery are more likely to resume normal sexual activity than are men who have had heart attacks. This may be because the partner of the heart attack victim is apprehensive about another attack. Some cardiologists say that if a man can climb a flight of stairs, he can safely have sex. It's best to check with your doctor.

Schemes or devices to overcome impotence are as old as history. Potions have been drunk, gods have been invoked, lotions have been applied, witchcraft has been employed, honey and spices have been blended—all for the purpose of having sex with an impressive erection. Stimulants—or hoped-for stimulants—ranged from carrots and peas, parsnips, and herbs to powdered animal horns and ground-up genitals. The rhinoceros population was almost decimated because of an Oriental belief in the aphrodisiac powers of powdered rhino horns. This belief still exists among some people, poachers still kill rhinos for horns worth $1,000 apiece, and the danger of extinction of the endangered animals remains very real.

Man's search for foolproof sexual fulfillment has literally covered the globe, as though there were some particular place where sexual shortcomings could be cured. Ponce de Leon discovered Florida while in quest of a fabled "fountain of youth," and that meant just one thing.

Now medical science has found answers that have nothing to do with potions, powders, or places. Instead, they are quite practical. One is an injection, the other is an implant.

The "erector injector" is a drug that will cause a penis to become erect for from one and a half to three hours, long enough to sustain intercourse. It is a new treatment for impotence, and has been effective with about 80 percent of the men on whom it has been used.

The drug is vasoactive, meaning it works on blood vessels, and is available only by prescription. It has been effective for patients with diabetes, heart or neurological problems, and for those who have had radical prostate surgery.

The patient himself injects the drug directly into his penis. This presents certain disadvantages: Instruction and counseling by a physician are required, and inexperienced patients could place the injection in the wrong place and scar the penis. Another interesting complication is that an injection erection may not fade after a few hours, in which case some doctor will get an emergency call.

The process is not yet fully accepted, and it is expensive, but it is less expensive than surgical implantation of a penile prosthesis. More follow-up with this technique is necessary to ascertain its practicality and safety.

Implants (there are several kinds) are substitutions that don't differ much in principle from that expedient remedy of very early automobile days when an inner tube just wouldn't hold air anymore, and there was no replacement. At that juncture, a desperate driver filled his tire with sawdust instead of air. Now we have the implant, and it works quite well.

Artificial tubes called *penile prostheses* are inserted into the penis to do the work of natural tubes (corpora cavernosa) which ordinarily fill with blood to create an erection. They fit precisely into the chambers and fill them completely. These prostheses have been developed within the past ten to fifteen years, and their success has expanded their use dramatically. Thousands are in use in the United States.

There are two types of prostheses, solid and inflatable.

Solid tubes, in pairs, are made of silicone rubber with or without metal inserts (but not enough metal to set off an airport detector). The implants remain rigid all the time, providing a perpetual erection as large and full as a normal erection. This has the advantage of preparedness but the disadvantage of being difficult to conceal in clothing. Some carry five- or ten-year guarantees!

Inflatable prostheses also come in two types. Both use hollow cylinders that may be inflated to erect positions by pumping up a self-contained sterile fluid.

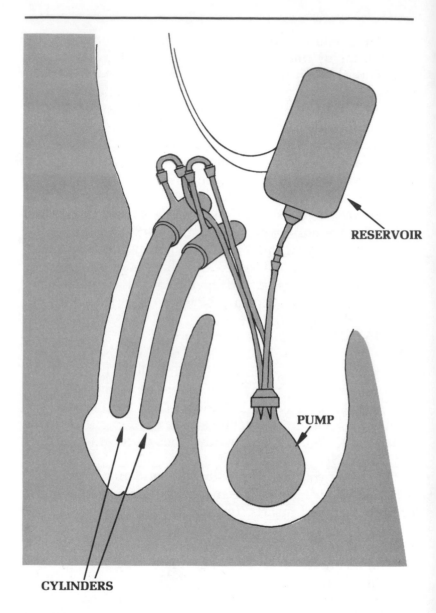

RESERVOIR

PUMP

CYLINDERS

Penile implant

In one type, fluid, reservoir, and pump all are carried within the cylinders themselves; erection is achieved by working the cylinder pumps. In the other type, fluid is held in a reservoir implanted in the abdomen and is forced into the cylinders by operating a pump implanted in the scrotum—all of this connected by a network of silicone tubing.

Implant operations for both solid and inflatable prostheses are now relatively routine. In fact, the solid implant may be performed on an outpatient basis; hospitalization overnight is required for an inflatable implant. In either case, sexual relations must be suspended until approved by a doctor, usually after four to six weeks. Other than slight postoperative discomfort for a short time, implants are popular and men have few complaints.

> Consider Charlie, whose job as a hotel night clerk gave him time to contemplate his troubles and the shortening of his life span. His troubles began (specifically, his sex life ended) with a cancer operation four or five years earlier. He read about penile prostheses, came in to ask about them, and decided to have one himself.
>
> He did nicely. I didn't see him again for weeks, and what I saw was a very changed Charlie. He had a spring in his step and a glint in his eye; he wore a loud sports jacket and a new hairstyle topped off with a jaunty tam.
>
> The psychological change was almost jarring. Charlie wasn't the same man, he was a cat. And there's no doubt about why. He bragged that he had entertained a lady friend and brought her to the first climax of her life after making love for forty-five minutes. He never could have done that without a prosthesis.

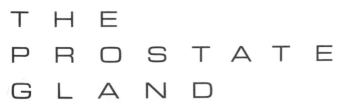

THE PROSTATE GLAND

I n a man's body, seminal fluid, or semen, is pumped under pressure to the penis to be discharged through ejaculation—after tiny tubes have added sperm to the seminal fluid mixture.

The prostate gland is a critical component of this process, and only males have it. But even to men, the prostate's function is obscure, its location vague, and its name often mispronounced (it's "prostate," not "prostrate").

The prostate is uniquely suited to perform critical male functions because of its composition and location. But a man can function without it, as we will see below.

Its composition is muscular and glandular.

Its location is immediately below the bladder, surrounding the tube that directs urine flow into the penis.

The muscular function, coordinated with muscles in the bladder, opens and closes the tube through which urine flows from the bladder to the penis. It also helps shut off urine at the bladder, permitting semen to enter the penis during periods of sexual arousal leading to ejaculation.

The glandular function of the prostate is to manufacture a portion of the semen—that sticky, milky seminal fluid that spurts through the penis during sexual orgasm.

The tube that carries both urine and semen through the penis is the urethra. Urine and semen cannot flow through the urethra at the same time. The prostate and bladder, with help from the brain and other stimuli, determine which it shall be.

These separate functions of the prostate are known and well understood. But much is still unknown about all the prostate does and how it works.

It is known that the prostate grows to its normal size, about the size of a walnut, at puberty. It enlarges again at about the age of fifty, a normal expansion related to aging. However, the prostate can expand well beyond its normal dimensions—in some cases it can grow as big as a grapefruit—for reasons that are not clear but are probably under hormone control. The excessive growth, called *adenoma*, is of a different tissue from normal prostate cells. As adenoma grows, it spreads inward and gradually applies increasing pressure to the urethra, as though a garden hose were gradually being pinched tight. When the urethra is partially pinched off, signs of prostate problems appear.

The body reacts to an enlarged prostate and a restricted urethra with plenty of symptoms. Almost all of them have to do with urination. Here are principal symptoms:

- Difficulty in urinating
- Changes in urinary habits, particularly more frequent urination at night
- Pain or a burning sensation while urinating
- Presence of blood in urine
- Irregular urine flow—a stream that starts, stops, stammers, and starts again
- Difficulty in stopping urine flow
- Persistent presence of dribbles that leave embarrassing spots on clothing

What's more, urination problems in the prostate can lead to related problems in other organs. For example, restricted urine flow in the prostate can put greater demands on the bladder and kidneys. This could lead to bladder infection and ultimately to kidney obstruction and failure, if unattended.

Another sign of potential prostate problems is pain that is not related to urination but is felt in other places. Pain in the lower back, pelvic region, or perineum is normal from time to time, but any pain that increases in frequency or intensity should be regarded as a warning. (The perineum is an area between the scrotum and the anus, that place most likely to be pinched by a small, narrow, or hard bicycle seat.)

Naturally, the earlier an enlarged prostate is detected, the greater is the chance that it can be corrected. The body provides some help, because the age when symptoms are likely to appear can be anticipated (it's usually after fifty), and the prostate itself is relatively easy to examine.

From an external perspective, the gland can be reached at its location in the rectum just inside the anus. In a routine digital ("finger wave") examination, a doctor can feel the prostate to test for irregularities or asymmetry (the prostate should be of normal size and a rubbery texture). The doctor's examination with a gloved, lubricated finger is painless and for most patients is only slightly uncomfortable. The examination is limited, however, because the doctor can feel only the back side of the gland, as though feeling the tip of an iceberg.

A new technique, called *transrectal ultrasonography,* can obtain more information about the prostate and may prove to be more effective in early detection of prostate cancer (which now is very hard to find in early stages). Ultrasonography works on the principle of sonar; it projects sound impulses back and forth across the prostate, working back layer after layer, and registers the reflected images on a screen like a TV set. Transrectal ultrasound examination of the prostate is not yet a proven prostate

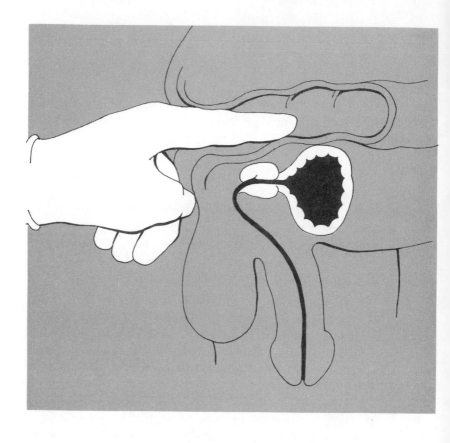

"Finger wave," or digital rectal examination, by way of the rectum to feel the prostate for problems such as cancer. Routine prostate examination should be performed at yearly intervals after the age of forty.

cancer screening technique. However, this technology does aid in guiding biopsy needles to suspicious areas of the prostate. Future studies are needed to determine its real potential.

The ultrasound machine usually is operated by a urologist, a specialist who deals with urinary-tract problems in men and women, and to whom a personal physician refers his patient if abnormalities are suspected.

PROSTATE PROBLEMS

Benign Prostatic Hyperplasia ["Old Man's Disease"]

Fred, a sixty-seven-year-old retired lumber broker, was getting up four to five times every night to urinate. He came to see me partly because he was worried but mostly because his wife was tired of being awakened by his frequent night calls.

Sometimes Fred's urine flow was normal, but at other times he was slow to start and slow to finish. He also felt the need to go again as soon as he got back in bed, but his return trips produced very little.

He said he had cut down on drinking, thinking that alcohol might have had something to do with his condition, but this didn't help much.

Fred said his father and two older brothers had had prostate operations. He wanted to know whether prostate conditions were hereditary, and I told him that we really don't know.

I did tell him that he needed a relatively simple operation to clear obstructive tissue *from his prostate. I performed a transurethral resection, the least complicated of prostate operations, and after a while Fred's urinating returned to normal. Now he gets up only once a night (some nights not at all).*

Fred's condition was benign prostatic hyperplasia, an apparent overproduction of cells within the prostate gland. Growth of adenoma tissue extends inward toward the urethra and in time can restrict urine flow and block the tube. A patient who was a logger described his condition nicely when he said, "Doc, I can't strip the bark off the tree anymore."

In addition to urination difficulties, some patients may experience pain with urination, or find blood in their urine but experience no pain.

Symptoms of this sort should be reported immediately to a doctor.

Acute Prostatitis ["Fire Below"]

Roger, aged twenty-eight, a professional basketball player, was overcome during a practice session with what seemed to be a sudden attack of flu. He had alternate chills and fever, muscular aches and pains all over, and discomfort in his lower back and perineum. Worse, he had to urinate frequently, and urination was very painful. At times his stream was pink, as if tinted with blood.

The team physician found that Roger's prostate gland was tender and swollen, and sent him to me. I diagnosed a urinary-tract infection (it was blood that Roger was seeing) and prescribed antibiotics and rest. Within a few days Roger felt only mild discomfort, and within a

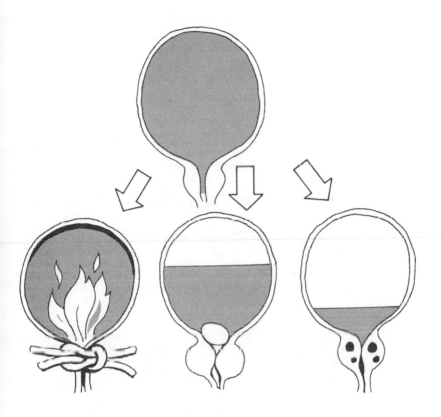

Three things that can happen to your prostate: Prostatitis, *left*, feels like a fire, with urinary frequency, burning, constriction, and possible bleeding caused by infection in most cases. Benign prostatic hyperplasia, *center*, is a normal benign growth that occurs with aging; the cause is unknown and symptoms include slow stream (flow), incomplete emptying, and urinary "blockage." Cancer, *right*, is also of an unknown cause; there may be no apparent symptoms present.

week he was back on the court. A subsequent examination revealed no further problems.

Acute prostatitis is an infection of the prostate gland caused by bacteria. It can occur in any man from adolescence to old age, and it often hits suddenly. Symptoms usually are a combination of urinary difficulties (as in hyperplasia) and nausea, chills, fever, vomiting, and aches and pains (as in influenza). Antibiotic drugs and rest are an effective treatment.

Chronic Prostatitis ["Pain Near the Ass"]

Malcolm, an engineer who plays golf where I do, confided in the locker room one day that he was having urinary-tract symptoms—the same symptoms that have shown every year or so for the last fifteen years. He had to urinate more often than usual, and felt a burning sensation each time he did so. Persistent symptoms brought him to the office.

He said he didn't have chills or fever, and saw no blood in his urine. Nevertheless, tests indicated a urinary-tract infection. I found he had low-grade prostatitis. Treatment was simple: I prescribed antibiotics and ordered him to take a warm bath two or three times a day. He could still play golf if he had time after all that.

Stress is frequently associated with chronic prostatitis, with or without a urinary-tract infection. It is a condition that professional men and business executives in high-stress jobs seem prone to acquire. So do truck drivers, who combine the stress of freeway driving with long periods of sitting in a bouncing cab. Antibiotics or urinary antiseptics are effective means of treatment.

Congestive Prostatitis ["Nothing Spells Relief"]

Reverend Smith, a forty-eight-year-old cele-bate clergyman, came in with pains in two hard-to-describe areas. One was perineal, which made him feel as if he had been riding a bicycle too long, and the other was suprapubic, which gave him a pain right below the navel. He said he also had to urinate frequently.

He confided that he had occasional dis-charges, usually white or clear, from his penis. He had no history of venereal disease, and no outlet for sex except occasional masturbation.

Reverend Smith's problem was congestion of the pros-tate. The congestion is caused by semen that clogs the tube because it hasn't been ejaculated. Frequent, urgent calls to urinate, often resulting in disappointing dribbles, are reported by males from adolescence on, particularly among single men and married men who are separated. Stress and other factors might be cited, but the clearly evident cause is a lack of sex. Doctors may prescribe sitz baths, massage, antibiotics, or whatever. The truth is that masturbation usually will clear the pipeline, just as a good blow will clear a stuffed-up nose.

Hematospermia ["Rusty Pipes"]

Marvin, aged sixty-seven, a retired accoun-tant, found blood on his pajamas one morning. It was just a few days after his wife reported blood in her vaginal discharge after having in-tercourse. A methodical man, Marvin deter-mined by masturbating who was doing the bleeding. Sure enough, his seminal fluid con-tained specks about the size and color of coffee grounds. That was when he came to me.

He had no pain, no blood in his urine, no other symptoms of hyperplasia. A complete urologic examination was normal. I told him not to worry, and come back in a year.

"Bloody come"—evidence of blood in ejaculate—is an alarming discovery for any man. The alarm can be compounded if his partner also finds blood coming from her body after intercourse.

What's happening usually is nothing worse than an inflammation of the prostate gland or seminal vesicles, which leaves traces of blood in semen. Or it could be that the excitement of intercourse and the fervor of ejaculation caused the eruption of a small blood vessel in one person or the other. The way to determine which person is bleeding is to do what Marvin did, masturbate and see.

Signs in the ejaculate usually appear in one of two shades, dark specks that resemble coffee grounds, or bright red stains. It is unusual for cancer to cause such bleeding, although "bloody come" is most likely to occur at a time of maximum vulnerability to cancers of the prostate and bladder.

Cancer of the Prostate ["Serious Business"]

Ralph, aged sixty-six, a businessman, told his doctor during a routine physical that he had to get up once or twice every night to urinate. He also said that drinking coffee or tea after dinner made things worse, so he quit. But for all the urgency, Ralph said his urine stream had slowed down in the past few years. Otherwise he was completely healthy; he had no indications of infection, bleeding, or backache, and his blood tests were normal.

After he was referred to me, I confirmed by

ultrasonic scanning that a small, one-half-inch nodule his doctor had discovered was in fact a firm spot on the right side of the prostate. Needle aspiration confirmed that the nodule was malignant, with a low-grade cancer of the prostate.

I performed a radical prostatectomy, which meant that I removed the entire prostate and the seminal vesicles that led to it, and reconnected the urethra directly to the bladder. Within a few weeks, Ralph returned to his regular daily routine. Eventually he was able to urinate normally, maintain erections, and have satisfactory intercourse. His cancer had been caught in time.

Bud, publisher of a well-respected small-town newspaper, announced to his readers that he would retire on his seventy-fourth birthday. What he didn't say was that he had cancer of the prostate.

Bud's symptoms were like those Ralph reported, some increased demands to urinate, but nothing more. Like Ralph, his tumor was discovered during a routine physical examination. Unlike Ralph—but like a discouraging majority of other men—his cancer was discovered after it had spread beyond the prostate.

Bud's cancer was inoperable; it was too late. He was subjected to "extensive and intensive" radiation, and his future beyond retirement is an unanswered question.

The statistics of prostate cancer are awesome. Prostate cancer is the second most fatal cancer among men, after lung cancer. It is responsible for 30,000 deaths in the

United States each year, and each year another 100,000 new cases of prostate cancer are diagnosed. Its incidence increases with age, and it is most prevalent between sixty and eighty years. It is not known when cancer of the prostate begins; after eighty, most men will have it but will not necessarily die of it. It is estimated that 30 percent of American men over age fifty will have cancer of the prostate. Using those figures, only 1 in 300 (1.4 percent) die of it!

Patients want to know if there are ways to protect against prostate cancer, and they often ask about theories they have heard. One theory holds that sexual activity is a deterrent. This always had been dismissed as wishful thinking, but a recent British study establishes some basis for the claim.

Other theories speculate on the relationships between diet and cancer or absence of cancer. It's all speculation; the answer is that there are no answers.

Cancer of the prostate is particularly insidious because it is difficult to detect; it reveals no identifiable signs in its early stages. Cancer might cause symptoms of obstruction as other prostate problems do, or it might show nothing at all. By the time cancer does leave possible clues—serious problems with urination, or persistent pain in the hip or back, for example—it may have spread beyond the prostate gland into neighboring bones, lymph nodes, and the bloodstream.

More than 90 percent of prostate cancer cases are inoperable when first seen by a urologist. However, if cancer is detected early, a majority of cases (85 percent) can be cured by surgical removal. After the age of forty, every man should have a prostate examination yearly.

If cancer has spread beyond the prostate, only treatment without a cure is possible. The options are not pleasant. One is to prescribe radiation therapy or chemotherapy; one is to administer estrogen, to neutralize the dominating effect of testosterone, which fuels the growth of prostatic cancer cells; one is to remove the testicles, source of testosterone, to slow the growth of cancer cells; and one is to do nothing. The fact that there are many long-term survivors after hormone treatment alone adds to the mysteries surrounding this disease. Because we don't know the natural history of cancer of the prostate, confusion exists as to the best treatment.

Any treatment, however, can do little but provide some relief and buy some time.

PROSTATE SURGERY

7

A common operation in the private parts department removes obstructions in the prostate gland that block or impede normal flow. A surgical instrument called a *resectoscope* enters the gland and cuts away blockage piece by piece.

The operation offers a safe and completely effective solution for men who seem to have to urinate all the time, or can't empty their bladders completely, or lose sleep because they must get up so often at night.

It is the answer for the fellow who misses the best part of the ball game because he's in the rest room under the stands trying to get something going at the urinal, the fellow who can hear the excitement and can't help but notice that two men and a boy have come and gone in the next stall while he's still standing in place.

The name for this operation is *transurethral resection of the prostate,* or TURP. It has become so common among older men that it now is one of the most frequently performed operations financed through Medicare. By the year 2000 it probably will be performed on one-third of the male population over age sixty-five in this country, partly because men are living longer while their parts are wearing out.

The name gives a clue to how the operation is performed. *Transurethral* means that the surgical instrument is directed through the urethra—the normal channel through the penis—to reach the prostate. No skin incision is necessary. This sounds gruesome, but the operation is painless and so is the postoperative period. For most patients, a hospital stay of two or three nights is all that is required. Because there is no incision, there is no scar to heal.

Symptoms that bring men into the doctor's office and that ultimately lead to a TURP operation ordinarily involve problems in passing urine. These can be an urgency to get up four or five times a night, difficulty in starting, pain during urination, inability to empty the bladder satisfactorily, a need to urinate again after having just done so, a urine flow that starts and stops, even dribbling on one's pants.

On examination, the doctor probably will find that the prostate feels somewhat enlarged. He may assist his diagnostic effort with an X ray of the kidneys or an ultrasound examination of the prostate. In most cases, the finding will be a condition called benign prostatic hyperplasia, an apparent overproduction of cells. The cause of hyperplasia is unknown but the result is a growth within the prostate that crowds against the urethra. Crowding impedes or blocks flow from the bladder and creates difficulties with urination, just as a clamp set too tight could cut off flow in a garden hose. The purpose of the operation is to remove the obstructing growth, like peeling an orange from the inside but leaving the rind or prostate unchanged.

The resectoscope, the instrument that is inserted through the penis, is a long metal tube with a light, a channel for water flow, and a loop of fine wire that can be charged with controlled amounts of electricity. The surgeon moves the loop back and forth, his hand motions akin to playing a tiny trombone, and chips away at the excess growth. The chips are irrigated out by water. The operation takes about an hour; as mentioned above, it is not painful and neither is the postoperative period. After the operation, a catheter is inserted through the prostate and into the bladder to drain blood and urine and give the bladder a rest.

Usually the patient can eat a normal meal on the evening after or on the morning following the operation. The catheter may be removed the following morning. Then the patient may go home, to lead a sedentary life for three to four weeks. The operation is successful in 95 percent of all cases; in a few cases, regrowth of obstructive tissues may occur.

Urinary incontinence is not common after a transurethral resection. There may be mild leakage for a time after returning from the hospital; this usually clears up after a few weeks. And in most cases the operation does not cause impotence (the inability to get an erection); if the patient was potent before the operation, he will usually be potent after it. However, there is a difference between impotence and sterility. Frequently, patients become infertile after a transurethral resection because the operation changes the structure of the bladder neck. That change, in turn, diverts ejaculate from its normal path through the penis, so that it goes into the bladder instead. There is no change in sensation, but at the moment of orgasm a man may be having a retrograde ejaculation—he is going instead of coming.

A TURP operation is not a guarantee against cancer; that is not its purpose. It is still possible that cancer unrelated to the operation can develop months or years later.

Every year thousands of men have the operation, and of course many of them like to talk about it. A man contemplating such an operation could profit by talking with those who have had the operation.

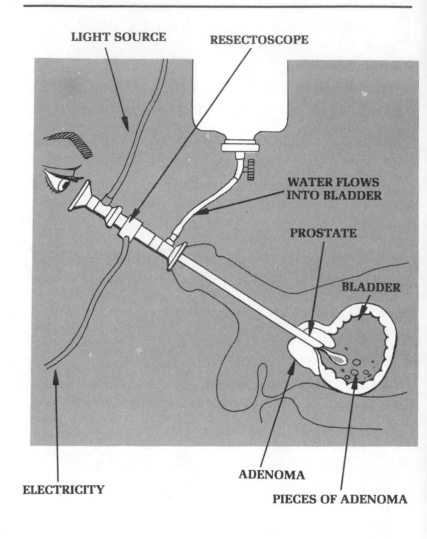

LIGHT SOURCE   RESECTOSCOPE

WATER FLOWS
INTO BLADDER

PROSTATE

BLADDER

ADENOMA

PIECES OF ADENOMA

ELECTRICITY

Transurethral resection of the prostate—a common operation
for obstruction in men, done through the normal channel, or
transurethrally.

RADICAL PROSTATECTOMY

If the transurethral prostatic resection is a minor tune-up, a radical prostatectomy is a major repair. It is the complete removal of the prostate, as compared with a resection that chips away obstructing growth.

A radical prostatectomy is the only effective cure for cancer of the prostate. Its potential is extremely limited, however, because surgery is effective only if the cancer is detected in its early stages. In fact, only a few cancer patients are candidates for a radical prostatectomy because in a majority of cases cancer has spread beyond the prostate before being discovered.

A radical prostatectomy removes not only the prostate but the pouchlike seminal vesicles behind it, both of which produce seminal fluid that carries sperm to and through the penis. A man who has had a radical prostatectomy may no longer father children.

Symptoms of prostatic cancer can be the same as those of an enlarged but noncancerous prostate, i.e., various problems with urination. But a doctor may also find a hard spot or bump on the side of the prostate during his routine digital examination, and that is a strong indication of cancer.

Cancer of the prostate is insidious—it may exhibit no symptoms at all. The way to diagnose the cancer is to take samples with a needle in either of two ways, *needle aspiration* or *needle biopsy*. Compare it with taking a sample of an apple; the needle can sample the juice (aspiration) or a piece of the pulp (biopsy).

If cancer is diagnosed, it is mandatory that the doctor determine the extent of cancerous growth. When cancer has spread beyond the prostate, no operation can cure it. Blood tests, a bone scan, and tests of lymph nodes are means used to estimate the extent and intensity of cancerous growth. If the cancer is quite active microscopically—

rating, say, eight on a scale of ten—an operation would not be recommended.

Until a few years ago, removal of the prostate meant the end of a satisfying sex life as well. But development of a "nerve sparing" technique by Dr. Patrick Walsh, chairman of the Department of Urology at the Johns Hopkins University School of Medicine in Baltimore, allows preservation of the nerves that touch off the sensation of orgasm. Both potency and the exhilaration of climax remain intact.

A radical prostatectomy requires open surgery, usually an incision from the belly button to the pubic bone above the penis. The operation takes two to three hours, and the normal hospital stay is from seven to ten days.

Cancer of the bladder requires removal of both the prostate and the bladder. The operation, called a radical cystoprostatectomy, is discussed in Chapter 9.

SEXUALLY TRANSMITTED DISEASES

8

Venereal diseases now have a new name, "sexually transmitted diseases." Some take new forms: AIDS is unprecedented and alarming; some, such as syphilis, recede from prominence; others, such as herpes and hepatitis B, which have been around for years, have caught popular attention. Whether they're called VD or STD, they're here to stay.

Listed below are America's most troublesome sexually transmitted diseases.

SYPHILIS

Syphilis ("syph," "gumma") has been around a very long time. It swept across Europe in the latter part of the fifteenth century and probably was brought to North America by the crew members of Columbus or of another explorer of his time. Syphilis has been in America since the continent was discovered.

Syphilis can be effectively cured if treated immediately with penicillin. But if it is untreated and allowed to reach its advanced stage—years after infection—it can cause paralysis, insanity, blindness, even death.

The bacteria that cause syphilis, spiral-shaped microorganisms called *Treponema pallidum*, are transmitted by sexual contact, by touching an infected sore, or direct contact with infected blood. They also can be transferred from a pregnant woman to her fetus.

If allowed to run its course, syphilis occurs in three stages:

Primary The first indication of syphilis is a chancre (pronounced SHANK-er) which appears about two to four weeks after infection. It begins as a dull red spot, then becomes a pimple, then ulcerates into a round or oval sore with a craterlike edge. This is the chancre. The sore is about the color of raw ham, is firm, and is neither tender nor painful. Even if untreated, it usually heals in three or four weeks, leaving the impression that the syphilis has gone away. This is part of syphilis's deception.

Secondary If the syphilis has been treated with penicillin, no doubt it will be cured. But if not, a second stage will follow at some time between a week and six months after the chancre has healed.

Symptoms of the second stage include a pale or pinkish rash on the palms of the hands and soles of the feet, fever, a sore throat, headaches, pains in the joints, hair loss, a poor appetite, and even weight loss. But the most serious symptoms are open sores that appear on the genitals and anus and are highly contagious.

Because of its variety of symptoms and signs that are characteristics of other diseases, syphilis is sometimes called the "great imitator" and is often diagnosed incorrectly. This is another aspect of its deception.

This second stage usually lasts three to six months, although it can recur periodically. Then all symptoms disappear and the syphilis seems to have gone away again. Instead, it has entered another dormant period. It is no longer contagious, but its infections enter and grow in other parts of the body.

Tertiary This is "late syphilis" that usually shows years after the first stage. It brings with it serious problems with the brain, spinal cord, eye, heart, or wherever the infections have been growing. Severe complications can cause insanity, paralysis, blindness, even death.

GONORRHEA

Gonorrhea ("clap," "drip") is the most common and oldest of sexually transmitted diseases. Moses was instructed to warn of its uncleanness in the Old Testament (Leviticus 15), and Plato, Aristotle, and Hippocrates mentioned it. Gonorrhea also is one of the most common infectious diseases. In the United States, more than a million cases are reported each year, but the actual number of new cases may be many times that.

Gonorrhea has a short incubation period, from one to eight days after infection. Its usual symptom is a yellowish discharge from the penis.

The transmission route is through sexual contact—intercourse, fellatio, anal intercourse. All these are sexual activities, but there is evidence that inanimate objects may also be involved. That old excuse, "I caught it on a toilet seat," was proven by me to be at least theoretically possible. My experiments showed that the bacteria in their natural state last as long as two hours on a toilet seat or wet toilet paper. Although this route of asexual transmission is rare, it is possible (*New England Journal of Medicine*, 301: 91–93, July 12, 1979).

Gonorrhea can be cured by penicillin. Some gonorrheal organisms may resist penicillin, however, and require an alternative drug.

A doctor known to be quite particular in his habits slipped off for a weekend in Nevada. He engaged a prostitute but insisted first that she show that she was free of herpes or AIDS. The lady apparently offered evidence to his satisfaction. However, when he got home he was clean of herpes and AIDS, all right, but had the clap.

VENEREAL WARTS

Venereal warts are growths that occur in cool, moist areas, particularly the penis, scrotum, and anus. They have a white, rough surface, something like a cauliflower, and grow singly or in clusters. They are painless and can be easily removed, but their ugly appearance could deter a potential sex partner. Warts may coexist with other sexually transmitted diseases, and are probably the most contagious of them all. The virus survives well outside the body.

GENITAL HERPES

Genital herpes is a viral-transmitted skin infection that affects some 20 million people, many of whom carry it for life because there is no known cure. Some individuals may have only one outbreak in a lifetime, but others may have many, often instigated by stress or depression.

The result is the appearance of small pimples that burn with pain. Some blisters appear singly, but most develop in clusters of ten to twenty on the penis, urethra, or rectum in men, and on the vaginal lips, cervix, or rectum in women. A tingling sensation may precede the pimples, and the first outbreak may be accompanied by a fever, headache, burning with urination, discharge from the penis, and swollen glands in the groin.

After a few days the headache and fever will fade away and the pimples will burst and form open sores. The sores will crust over and heal in about two weeks, leaving the patient with the impression that the herpes has gone.

Instead, the herpes virus will have moved into a dormant stage and, in 90 percent of cases, will strike again. The time of the next attack and the pattern of subsequent attacks vary from a few weeks to many years. Recurrent attacks may be stimulated by emotional distress, physical exhaustion, illness, sunburn, or may appear for no evident reason at all.

Subsequent attacks are likely to be less severe because the body is prepared for them, and their timing may vary considerably, but herpes almost always comes back.

Phil is a fellow who has been known to play around a little. One night—early in the morning, really—he called from a resort out of town. He said he had an emergency, and his voice was high-pitched with fear. The emergency was that he'd found an attractive lady in the bar and they had gone to his room for sex. After they were finished, she announced something like, "Oh, by the way, I have herpes. I thought you'd like to know."

Phil held out some hope for himself. He had used a condom, so he wanted to be assured that a condom was protection against herpes. I had to tell him it was not. A condom provides protection where it blocks direct contact with a herpes sore, but it is of no help if a sore is anywhere else.

CRABS

Pubic lice ("crabs") are parasites that attach themselves to pubic hair, are quite prevalent, and require fresh blood daily—they must bite to live. They are small, white, oval-shaped bugs, but under a microscope they look like translucent ocean crabs.

Crab lice are transmitted during sexual contact, "hair to hair." Although they are most prevalent in pubic hair, crabs can leap to eyebrows and eyelashes during fellatio or cunnilingus. They also can be acquired from sheets, towels, or clothing used by an infected person.

A week will pass before crabs begin to itch, but a reinfection (crabs are constantly hungry) will be evident within a day. Crab lice can survive only twenty-four hours after they leave the human body, but their eggs can survive up to six days in sheets or clothing.

Although crabs are an irritant, infestation is not a serious disease. A few people feel no symptoms, but most develop an itchy rash that can become infected.

An effective way to get rid of crabs is to apply a chemical, 1 percent gamma benzene hexachloride, which is available as a lotion or shampoo marketed under the trade name Kwell. Kwell lotion applied to pubic hair must be left on for twenty-four hours; Kwell shampoo should be rubbed into all hairy areas vigorously for ten minutes before being rinsed off. The shampoo treatment should be repeated in a week if any nits (crab eggs) remain. Eyelash infestation must be treated by applying petroleum ophthalmic ointment twice daily for ten days.

An assistant in a congressman's office was attracted to a woman on the staff, but always felt she was unapproachable. She was blond, bright, and pretty and always pleasant, but the fellow felt intimidated by her vaguely distant airs. He had never dared ask her for a date.

One evening after an office party he threw caution to the wind and invited her to his place for another drink. She accepted and, to his surprise, spent the night with him. About a week later he was further surprised to discover his first case of crabs.

HEPATITIS B

Hepatitis B is one of many forms of viral hepatitis, a liver infection that can cause chills, fever, diarrhea, nausea, anorexia (the need to vomit), and possibly jaundice (a liver condition which turns the skin yellowish.) Extreme consequences can be chronic liver disease and/or death.

Hepatitis B virus is transmitted through blood, saliva, seminal fluid, vaginal secretions, and other body fluids. Approximately 200,000 active cases are diagnosed annually in the United States, some of them sexually transmitted. Additionally, up to four times as many people may be hepatitis carriers, those who are infected with the disease but are not ill from it.

There is no known cure for hepatitis B, so the only treatment is supportive—intended to make the patient feel better. A vaccine has been developed to act as a preventative, but it is not effective after the disease has been acquired.

MOLLUSCUM CONTAGIOSUM

Molluscum contagiosum is a painless skin lesion, a small pinkish or orange bump that, when squeezed, will pop a plug of material similar to a blackhead. It appears on the genitalia, thighs, buttocks, and lower abdomen. It does not cause much trouble and it often disappears, even without treatment, over a period of months.

CHANCROID

Chancroid is a sexually transmitted disease rare in the United States but common in the tropics. If your partner has been in a tropical climate, check with your doctor.

NONSPECIFIC URETHRITIS

Nonspecific urethritis (NSU) represents a category of relatively minor but rapidly spreading sexually transmitted diseases. Their common symptoms—discharge from the penis and pain while urinating—are also common to gonorrhea, but NSUs are "non-gonococcal," meaning non-gonorrheal. In fact, they resist treatment by penicillin, the usual cure for gonorrhea.

Chlamydia, one of the NSU group, is the most prevalent sexually transmitted disease in the United States. Tetracycline is usually an effective treatment. If chlamydia is left untreated, secondary infections can reach other organs and result in infertility.

The initials NSU seem less accusatory than the word "gonorrhea," and for that reason NSU frequently appears on medical records. In the military, for example, it has happened often enough that officers and enlisted men have gone to town and done the same things, probably with the same women, and returned to the base with the very same infections. Officers' records would note presence of some NSU, but enlisted men's records would report infection by gonorrhea. The officers had the clout and the enlisted men had the clap.

AIDS

AIDS (acquired immune deficiency syndrome) was first reported in the United States in 1981, and there is good evidence that the number of cases is increasing each year. The disease breaks down the body's protective immune system, leaving it vulnerable to serious disease. The disease has reached epidemic status in the United States and worldwide. There is no known cure.

AIDS is caused by a human immunodeficiency virus (HIV) that is transmitted by sexual activity or by specific other means, such as transfusion of contaminated blood or use of contaminated drug paraphernalia. How AIDS is sexually transmitted—or not transmitted—is a subject of much misunderstanding. Perhaps this definition of transmission may help:

> *Any sexual activity involving exposure to the blood, semen, or vaginal secretions of an HIV-infected person can result in AIDS virus transmission.*

Although there is no known cure, the proper use of a condom and avoidance of certain sexual practices can reduce the risk of AIDS considerably.

Questions frequently asked are: How do I know if I don't have AIDS? How do I know that my sexual partners in the past ten to fifteen years did not have AIDS?

The high-risk AIDS group includes homosexual and bisexual men, intravenous drug users, and transfusion recipients. It includes men who have been involved with prostitutes or with women who are IV drug users or have had other sexual partners in the high-risk group.

If a patient is truly concerned about the possibility of having AIDS, I recommend that he undergo a blood test, especially if he is in a high-risk category. A positive test result indicates infection with the HIV virus, but not necessarily with the disease AIDS itself.

Antibodies to the AIDS virus will appear in a blood test from three weeks to six months or longer after a person has been infected. Medical science does not yet know how many years after exposure a person may still be at risk for a full-blown onset of the disease. If you feel you must be tested, see your physician or call the AIDS toll-free hot line, 1-800-342-AIDS (7514). At this time in the United States, most physicians are not trained to give AIDS information.

There are different types of tests for antibodies, but the

results may be misleading. The Enzyme-Linked Immu-
noabsorbent Assay (ELISA) has been known to give false
positive readings; that is, inaccurate positive results. The
Western Blot Test is used to confirm the positive ELISA
test. New tests are being developed that may prove to be
more accurate.

T H E
B L A D D E R

9

Nature arranged the working parts of a human urinary system from top to bottom in a logical order to perform separate but related functions.

At the top are the kidneys, which process urine and pass it through tubes, called *ureters*, down into the bladder. There urine is held until its release through a tube with a slightly different name, the urethra. As mentioned previously, in a man's body, the urethra passes through the prostate gland, which is immediately below the bladder neck, and through the penis to exit the body.

Unlike other parts of the system, the bladder has only one function. It is a reservoir to hold and release urine. Its capacity is twelve to fifteen ounces, about equal to the volume of a can of beer.

Because of their proximity, prostate and bladder functions are closely related and problems of the prostate often become problems of the bladder.

Obstructions or blockage of the prostate put pressure on bladder muscles, which must work harder to evacuate urine. The muscles begin to thicken and enlarge, just as biceps in the upper arm build up with heavy use. The thickening can reduce bladder capacity, requiring urination more frequently than normal.

Or pressure from the prostate may have an opposite effect, causing bladder muscles to stretch instead of thicken. This usually occurs after long-term blockage in the prostate. The distended bladder holds more urine than it should, and does not empty completely with each voiding; only the top of the reservoir goes and most of the urine remains. The bladder is constantly almost full, and usually feels full.

> A seventy-year-old farmer came in to see me about his expanding girth, although he probably wouldn't have come at all if his wife hadn't wondered why she had to let out his pants so often to relieve pressure around his abdomen.
>
> I asked him about his urinary habits. He said he spent long hours on his tractor and had trained himself to hold back his bladder so he wouldn't have to stop work to urinate.
>
> I found he had a greatly distended bladder and drained more than a quart of urine, more than twice the normal amount. I then did a transurethral resection of his prostate to clear up a related problem.
>
> Now he is able to empty his bladder normally, and his girth has returned to its size of five years ago. He's back to smaller clothing, and he feels more comfortable. He might be even more comfortable than that, because he gave farm and tractor to his son and drove his air-conditioned Cadillac to Palm Springs, where he and his wife bought a retirement condominium.

Among other results from stretching are *diverticula*, which are pouches or bubbles that distend from weak points on bladder walls. The bubbles, large or small, form when the bladder is under pressure, just as a weakened lining in an inner-tube wall swells disproportionately when the tube is inflated.

FLOW METER CHECKUP

Here is a way you can check your own urine flow rate to see whether it is adequate, and therefore normal. All it requires is a measuring cup and a watch with a second hand.

With a full bladder, begin urinating. When the stream becomes full, urinate into the cup for ten seconds, then move the cup away. Normal urine flow is 20 cubic centimeters a second (the range is 15–25 cc), so if your cup holds 200 cc (7 or 8 ounces) after ten seconds, you're right on the mark. If it holds noticeably less, see your doctor. If it holds more, that's fine. Another simple test is to write your initials in the snow.

Incidentally, certain foods cause changes in the urine of some men. An apparent bloody tinge may show up after eating beets. The color is due to the presence of Betanin, a red pigment, not blood cells. Beeturia is often misinterpreted as bloody urine by the unsuspecting.

The pungent urinary odor produced by some individuals within a short time after eating asparagus can also be alarming. It is debatable whether the latter condition is a problem with how the body handles the chemistry in asparagus or is a sensitivity to the odor. These strange happenings are nothing to worry about.

Another bladder condition, fortunately rare, is *interstitial cystitis*. It is characterized by low bladder capacity, bladder pain, and frequent voiding—as often as three or four times an hour, five to ten times a night. The filling bladder often triggers severe pain which can only be relieved by urination. The cause is not known, but close inspection reveals in most cases the existence of a bladder ulcer.

More familiar bladder problems include inflammation, stones, and cancer. Inflammation of the bladder is often associated with inflammation of the prostate and usually can be treated with antibiotics.

Stones are deposits of uric acid or calcium, something like deposits of scale in a radiator, and are caused by an obstruction of the prostate or mishandling of chemicals by the body. Stones can be passed naturally or be removed either mechanically or electrically.

The lining cells of the kidneys, the bladder, and the ureter connecting them all are of the same type. Cancer can develop in any of these, but the most common location is the bladder. Cigarette smoking, so often identified with lung cancer, also has been incriminated as a possible source of cancer of the bladder because of a reaction between chemicals in cigarette smoke and lining cells in the urinary tract. A significant sign is blood in the urine. It is "painless bleeding," but it is a danger sign.

> A chef, aged forty-four, came in after painless bleeding for three consecutive days. He had no prior experience with bleeding, was otherwise healthy, and his physical examination was normal. He admitted to smoking two packs of cigarettes daily for twenty-five years.
>
> X rays revealed normal kidneys but an abnormal mass in his bladder. The mass was malignant, and I removed it with a resectoscope. The tumor was non-infiltrating, which meant that its roots were not so deeply embedded in the bladder as to prevent complete removal. Bladder tumors tend to recur, however, so close observation with regular follow-up was mandatory. The patient also was advised to quit smoking, and he did.

Ruptures of the bladder or the urethra often occur in automobile accidents if the bladder is full. After an accident, a trouble sign that mandates immediate attention is either the presence of blood in the urine or no urine output. As a precaution, anybody about to travel in a car should empty his bladder first. An empty bladder doesn't rupture, but a full bladder can burst like a ripe melon.

> The emergency room reported the arrival of a man by ambulance one evening after a passing motorist found him in his overturned car off a county road. Examination determined that, among other things, the man had a ruptured bladder and a badly fractured pelvic bone. Ragged edges from the broken bone tore the bladder wall, so that the bone intended to protect the bladder was adding to its injuries.
>
> Later the man said he couldn't remember when he had last urinated. What happened was urine had leaked into his abdomen, a very dangerous situation.

A cystoscope is a surgical instrument that resembles a miniature telescope, with a long extension for insertion up the penis through the urethra. It also has a water supply and fiber-optic light source and is capable of exploring the entire urinary tract—urethra, prostate, and bladder. With a smaller attachment, a doctor can examine the kidneys for stones, tumors, or other abnormalities.

A similar instrument, a resectoscope with special attachments, can remove bladder stones in several ways—mechanically, electrically, or ultrasonically. It can disintegrate stones from the size of peas to golf balls and flush out debris through the penis. No incision is required. Also, most bladder cancers can be removed with a resectoscope.

However, if cancerous tumors are found to be infiltrating the bladder wall, growing like weeds, more drastic measures are necessary. An operation can remove the prostate and the bladder. In this extreme case, a segment of the small bowel is transplanted to serve as a reservoir—a small bladder joined directly to the kidneys, using ureters as urine conduits. Urine is drained from the substitute bladder into a small bag glued to the skin outside the body.

A young man who had just entered Britain's diplomatic service was assigned to routine chores at an international conference where Winston Churchill was present. At one fortunate moment he found himself alone with the great statesman.

Taking advantage of the opportunity, he asked Churchill for any advice appropriate for a young man entering His Majesty's diplomatic service.

Churchill pursed his lips for a moment, then said, "Young man, never pass up the opportunity to take a leak."

THE HARD FACTS: QUESTIONNAIRE RESULTS

10

Mike, a patient of mine, has a small garage where he has repaired all kinds of cars for all kinds of drivers during forty years in business. He has followed transmission trends from stick shifts to automatics, and back to stick shifts; he has nursed hand throttles, automatic chokes, and fuel injectors.

Just as Mike has kept up with changes in cars, he has adjusted to changes in drivers. Some complain about the slightest squeak, while others nurse the old buggy as long as it will stay on the road; some know absolutely nothing about a car, others volunteer diagnoses whether they're right or wrong.

Mike knows his customers and has concluded that drivers are like cars; all are similar, yet each is different. He might find his hunches confirmed in a survey I conducted to determine lifestyles and sex styles of one hundred men—in this case business and professional men who have achieved success in their thirty-five to fifty years of life. Many had advance degrees, and all were affluent, more than half earning at least $175,000 a year. Three-fourths of them were married, with two or three children. Ninety-six percent said they were heterosexual. Thirty-five percent had had vasectomies.

They were assured that the survey would be confidential and that their personal results would be disclosed only to them.

Most claimed some church attendance (53 percent were Protestant, 21 percent Catholic, and 7 percent Jewish).

These gentlemen reported—with anonymity and with nobody looking over their shoulders—they couldn't find much change in their sexual appetites and sexual prowess in the years since they were twenty-five, they enjoyed and encouraged oral sex with their wives or girlfriends, and that intercourse was still the best way to go, though for some it now took longer.

Almost all men questioned were married or had been, and a third of those currently married admitted having sexual affairs. The number of extramarital partners ranged from one to an impressive, if credible, ninety-eight. Apparently, they think marital fidelity is more essential for wives than for themselves, because 82 percent of the husbands thought their wives were faithful.

Only one of these fellows acknowledged having lost all interest in sex; the others stayed keyed up. They rated appearance as the major attraction in the opposite sex, and the looks they were looking for translated into breasts and buttocks—the formula that ignites fires in male imaginations.

Here is what the study has revealed:

HEALTH

This was a healthy group. Most claimed health that was excellent or above average. Perhaps because they were feeling good, only one-third got annual physical examinations—some only because their companies or their wives required them. Another third went to a doctor only when they were sick, and a few said going to a doctor didn't do any good.

None had had a heart attack, two-thirds exercised with some regularity—some vigorously, some languidly—and more than half said they maintained a healthy diet, had cut down on consumption of red meat, and had reduced salt intake in the past few years.

Some (13 percent) had high blood pressure, a possible cause of impotence, but only 4 percent took medication for hypertension. One in four reported a family history of diabetes, and two thirds said the health problem they feared most was cancer.

Drinking was out completely for three of every ten respondents. More (60 percent) drank two to four ounces a day, whether hard liquor, wine, or beer, and 10 percent drank more than four ounces a day. Only one in ten said he drank alcohol at a business lunch.

Most (88 percent) did not smoke cigarettes.

Perhaps because they enjoyed good health, very few acknowledged being too tired to do things. Almost all enjoyed job positions with authority and were satisfied with their careers, and every one (100 percent) felt good about his future.

MARRIAGE

Just 5 percent of these men were single. The others were in various stages of matrimony: married (78 percent), divorced (15 percent), or separated (2 percent). Of those who were married, 72 percent had married once, 23 percent twice, and 5 percent three or more times. Most had two or three children.

Most husbands judged that their lives with their wives were pleasurable (44 percent) or very pleasurable (44 percent). When asked in more specific terms, they offered these results, still generally favorable: Half reported a "central satisfaction" with life lived with their mates, and

19 percent said they vitally shared everything with their wives. But 12 percent conceded conflict or controlled tension (albeit "discreet and polite"), 9 percent admitted that marriage had dulled in middle age, and 7 percent acknowledged dull and routine marriages with emphasis on other things.

Every husband said communication with his wife was important. The subjects most frequently mentioned were money, children, and use of leisure time. About eight men in ten said that they were comfortable discussing sex with their wives, and that conversation often starts in the kitchen.

Each executive was asked to identify his best friend, and more than half named their wives. More than a third would go first to their wives for personal advice (best friends were second, chosen by 22 percent). One man in five had considered divorce (usually he was deterred because of the children). Fewer than half (41 percent) of married men wore wedding rings.

EXTRAMARITAL AFFAIRS

One-third of these husbands acknowledged having had an affair. Specifically, 34 percent admitted having extramarital intercourse, 61 percent denied it, and 4 percent said it wasn't applicable, whatever that means. One bachelor said he was having an affair, presumably cheating on his girlfriend.

Some (17 percent) said they had patronized prostitutes in the previous five years.

Answers to the fidelity question varied according to the number of marriages experienced by a respondent. Each was asked to respond to this question regarding his present marital relationship. Among once-married men, 40 percent acknowledged affairs; among twice-married,

22 percent, and among the few married three or more times, two-thirds admitted having had affairs. Evidently these fellows had given up on marriage as an institution.

Asked how many other women they had had during their marriages, most husbands ranged between one and five. About 20 percent said one only, but one prodigious fellow claimed to have slept with ninety-eight women. Most of these fellows liked extracurricular affairs; 85 percent rated them pleasurable or very pleasurable.

Were wives playing the same game? Presumably not. Only 10 percent of the husbands knew their wives were cheating, or thought they were, and 82 percent trusted their wives. Did the women know about their men? The conjecture among husbands was split, fifty-fifty.

PERFORMANCE

Most men said they had sexual intercourse from one to four times a week; one-third said twice a week. Only 4 percent reported no sex at all during a week.

When does all this happen? It appears that ten o'clock on Saturday night is a poor time to call the boss. Saturday night is still the action night (cited by 43 percent of respondents), and ten o'clock is happy hour (a choice of 45 percent). Other preferred days were Sundays and Fridays; the second favored hour was the next morning.

Who does the arousing? Men get things started, or think they do, on about two-thirds of all occasions; men and women initiate sex together the other third of the time. But very seldom does a wife initiate sex herself. This arrangement seemed satisfactory to only about 60 percent of those surveyed; the rest said things might be better if wives initiated sex more frequently.

Nearly all men surveyed (92 percent) had performed cunnilingus and most (85 percent) enjoyed applying it.

Three-fourths of the men enjoyed fellatio, but only half thought their wives liked it too. Oral sex often served as a preliminary to intercourse.

Once intercourse began, a substantial majority of the men (93 percent) said they achieved orgasm every time or almost every time. The rest claimed orgasm about three-fourths of the time.

About one-fourth of them (23 percent) said they thought their mates climaxed three-quarters of the time; twice as many men (46 percent) surmised that their partners reached orgasm half the time.

Half the men claimed they could climax in two to five minutes; a very few (2 percent) said they had to work fifteen minutes to half an hour. Most (88 percent) had only one orgasm a night, but 10 percent said they could come twice, and a very few (2 percent) asserted they could come three times.

Some men conceded that it didn't always come out the way they'd have liked. More than half (59 percent) admitted they had failed to achieve or maintain an erection. The causes, in order cited, were being too tired, having too much to drink, or being with a new partner for the first time. A few men (18 percent) admitted having a different problem: premature ejaculation. And, surprisingly, 15 percent said they had faked orgasm at one time or another.

Men think and dream about sex—84 percent of those surveyed, at least. But our respondents reported that nocturnal erections and wet dreams became rarer as they grew older, and half of them said they didn't have wet dreams anymore.

LOST YOUTH

If these fellows answered their questions accurately, they hadn't lost a whole lot from their sexual prime time, back when they were twenty-five years old. By almost two to one, they claimed it didn't take them any longer to get an erection now than it had at age twenty-five, that they didn't require any more penile stroking to reach orgasm than in those heydays, and that the volume of ejaculate spurting from those erections was as much as it ever was. By three to one, they claimed their penises got as stiff as before and stayed stiff during sex. The big admitted loss, from those days of youth, was rejuvenation—three fourths conceded it did take longer to get another erection after orgasm than it once had.

Practically every respondent said he was easily or very easily aroused sexually, just as he had been at age twenty-five. Half said sex was more enjoyable. The opposite was true for masturbation, for 75 percent said they masturbated less frequently than they had at age eighteen—although 6 percent said they masturbated more.

Almost all men (95 percent) claimed their erections were as big as they ever were, and that they rose without pain. A few noticed that their penises would bend, and a few more (11 percent) said they had ejaculated without erections. As a matter of fact, both occurrences are normal.

Not that anything could be done about it, but each respondent was asked, just for fun, if he'd like to have a larger, more formidable penis. Given this choice, one-third of them said they'd like their erections another inch longer, please, and one in four would prefer another inch in circumference. Perhaps it is more significant that all the others were satisfied with their present dimensions. Maybe that was because only 18 percent of the men thought their wives or girlfriends would welcome a larger erection, and only 18 percent hoped to encounter a tighter vagina.

Something can be done about creating erections artificially (as described earlier, surgical implantation of penile prostheses can remedy the situation) if natural erection fails. Half the men questioned said they would favorably consider such an operation if matters came (or didn't come) to that. The answers indicate that acceptance of artificial devices has increased significantly in the last several years.

A few questions near the end of the lengthy survey, reached after the responding executives had put a good deal of time and thought into their answers, disclosed how much these fellows really were interested in sex.

Dominating answers to a multiple-choice question about ways to improve sex life were appeals for "more": more frequent intercourse—64 percent; the partner should initiate sex more often—40 percent; more frequent oral sex—46 percent; more spontaneous sex—40 percent.

Finally, the men were given a chance to get away from it all by checking off their favorite extracurricular activities. Sex was the second most popular activity, named by 16 percent of the respondents. Leading the list, the choice of 22 percent, was golf.

PERSONAL EQ: ERECTILE QUOTIENT QUIZ

11

A personal inventory of sexual impotence risks:

		Yes	No
1.	I have sugar diabetes.	—	—
2.	I have high blood pressure (hypertension).	—	—
3.	I take medication for high blood pressure.	—	—
4.	I smoke cigarettes.	—	—
5.	I take medication for heart irregularity.	—	—
6.	I find that I am too tired to do anything, and the future seems hopeless.	—	—
7.	My present weight is more than ten pounds over my ideal weight.	—	—
8.	I am happy with my career choice.	—	—
9.	I am satisfied with my mate.	—	—
10.	My daily diet is best described as balanced.	—	—
11.	In the last few years I have decreased red meat consumption in my diet.	—	—
12.	I am satisfied with my sexual variety.	—	—
13.	My erection has shown no change compared to my earlier years.	—	—

14. My erection has shown some change   __   __
    compared to my earlier years.

15. My penis is as firm and hard as it was in   __   __
    the past.

	a	b	c

16. I drink alcohol in this amount: __   __   __
    a. more than 2 oz. a day
    b. up to 2 oz. a day
    c. none

17. My exercise program is best described   __   __   __
    as:
    a. none
    b. mild or regular
    c. vigorous

18. I need more stimulation to get an   __   __   __
    erection, compared to earlier years:
    a. big change
    b. some change
    c. no change

19. After ejaculation, it takes me longer to   __   __   __
    get another erection, compared to
    earlier years:
    a. yes
    b. some change
    c. no change

20. My interest in sex, compared to earlier   __   __   __
    years, is:
    a. less strong
    b. same
    c. stronger

Key to Personal EQ

Questions 1–7: 0 points for each Yes; 10 points for each
 No.
Questions 8–15: 10 points for each Yes; 0 points for each
 No.
Questions 16–20: For each question, if your response was
 a., give yourself 0 points; if b., 5 points; if c., 10 points.

Add up your total points. The average score is 125. If your
score is 100 or below, consult your doctor.

Executive Lifestyle Survey
ERECTILE QUOTIENT DISTRIBUTION

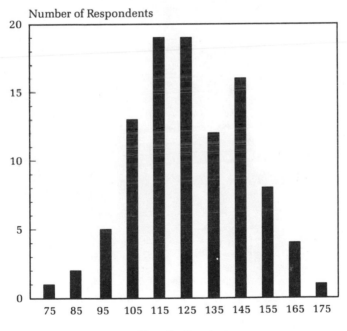

Erectile Quotient

RANGE: 75–175
MEAN: 129

PERSONAL UQ: URINATING QUOTIENT QUIZ

12

A personal inventory of bladder habits:

	Yes	No
1. I get up more than once a night to urinate.	—	—
2. My urine stream is slow, weak, and hesitant to start.	—	—
3. My urine flow is no longer steady; it stops, stutters, starts again.		—
4. I feel pain when I empty my bladder.	—	—
5. I see blood when I empty my bladder.	—	—
6. I have recurrent infection of the prostate.	—	—
7. I have had bladder stones in the past.	—	—
8. I dribble in my pants after I have zipped up.	—	—
9. Sometimes I feel like my urine flow is going to stop completely.	—	—
10. I have an aching feeling, with fever and chills, and difficulty emptying my bladder.	—	—

If you answer "yes" to any of these questions, see Chapter 6 for more information and consult your physician.

S E X
H I N T S

13

PLAY A LITTLE. Don't be short on foreplay. Being too eager is probably the number-one problem of most men. Men who take their time get the results.

TALK ABOUT IT. Tell your mate what you like and ask her what she likes best. Don't worry so much about whether you or she will have an orgasm. The "big O" will happen when it happens.

ENJOY YOURSELF. Sex should be fun, not a race or a performance goal.

SLOW DOWN. You miss a lot of scenery when you drive too fast down a country road. Set the stage yourself: devote more time to sex play.

TAKE TURNS. A lot of men complain that women are too passive. They could help by trading off and encouraging the woman to take turns being the aggressor.

BATHE. Even if you have a long-term mate, don't neglect personal hygiene. A shower or bath before sex will make it nicer for you both.

DON'T WORRY ABOUT SIZE. Men worry more than

women do about the size of their penis. You might be surprised to find that a compact model will do as well as a larger version. And if you have a larger version, be careful and considerate with your partner.

CHECK ALL BODY PARTS. Pay loving attention to other parts of her body—feet, legs, hands, back—as well as her breasts and other erotic areas.

LEARN TO LAUGH. The ability to laugh at yourself or the situation is very important. Laughter defuses tension, especially in a state of failure.

PRAISE. Make her feel special and she will make you feel special.

TAKE A VACATION. Rest and relaxation help, this time and the next time.

KEEP HEALTHY. Exercise and diet are important to keep your body in condition. The American Cancer Society recommends common sense and nutrition. Research is underway to evaluate and clarify the role of diet in the development of cancer. So far no direct cause-effect relationship has been proven, but we do know that some things you eat may increase or decrease your risks for certain types of cancer. Based on evidence at hand, you may lessen your chances for getting cancer by following these simple guidelines:

- Avoid obesity (twenty pounds over recommended weight for your height and age). Sensible eating habits and regular exercise will help to avoid excessive weight gain.
- Cut down on total fat intake. Eat less fat food to control your body weight more easily.

- Eat more high-fiber foods such as cereals, fresh fruit, and vegetables.
- Include foods rich in vitamins A and C in your daily diet. Choose dark green and deep yellow fresh vegetables and fruit (carrots, spinach, sweet potatoes, peaches, and apricots) as a source of vitamin A. Oranges, grapefruit, strawberries, and green and red peppers are rich in vitamin C.
- Include cruciferous vegetables in your diet. These include cabbage, broccoli, Brussels sprouts, kohlrabi, and cauliflower.
- Minimize salt-cured, smoked, and nitrite-cured foods. The American food industry has changed to new processes thought to be less hazardous.
- Drink alcohol only moderately and avoid smoking cigarettes.

Bladder—A reservoir for urine.

Epididymis—An elongated pouch on the back of the testicle where sperm mature.

Glans penis—The head of the penis.

Impotence—Inability to get an erection and maintain it through intercourse.

Penile prosthesis—An artificial substitute for a penile erection.

Penis—The male sexual organ, six inches long—more or less—when erect.

Perineum—The space between anus and back of the scrotum (where a bicycle seat hits your bottom).

Prostate gland (not "prostrate")—A male organ that surrounds the neck of the bladder and the urethra and produces some seminal fluid.

Prostatectomy—Surgical removal of the entire prostate gland (radical prostatectomy) or a portion of it (transurethral resection). See *TURP*, below.

Prostatitis—Inflammation of the prostate gland.

Scrotum—The sack that covers the testicles.

Semen (seminal fluid, ejaculate)—A thick, whitish secretion from male reproductive organs.

Seminal vesicles—Paired pouches behind the prostate that produce most of a man's seminal fluid.

Testicles—Male gonads that produce sperm and hormones.

Testosterone—A male sex hormone produced in the testicles.

TURP (transurethral resection of the prostate)—A surgical operation that removes growths within the prostate but spares the gland, comparable to removing pulp in an orange but leaving the rind.

Urethra—The tube that runs from the bladder through the penis to convey urine and seminal fluid.

Urethritis—An inflammation of the urethra.

Urologist—An investigator of a man's private parts.

Vas deferens—Tubes that carry sperm from the epididymis to ejaculatory ducts in the prostate.

Vasectomy—An operation that severs the vas deferens (see above) to render a man sterile.

I N D E X